Praise for *12 Questions for Love*

"I've known Topaz for over a decade, and *12 Questions for Love* is a perfect example of the incredibly curious, open, and uniting person behind {THE AND}. These seemingly simple questions distill years of observations, encouraging us to discuss what matters most and allow our relationships to thrive. Empowering and insightful, with heartfelt solutions to real-life problems, this is the book I wish I could've given to my younger self."

—**JODIE WHITTAKER**, actor

"In today's info-saturated world, answers are easy to come by—but powerful, connective questions are what we need more than ever. In this game-changing book, inspired by his award-winning film series, Topaz Adizes shares a dozen questions that can deepen and enrich the most important relationships in your life. Buy this book not just for yourself, but for the people you truly care about."

—**WARREN BERGER**, bestselling author of *A More Beautiful Question*

"Save yourself another round of heartbreak and breakups and *read this first*. Topaz condenses years of wisdom into 12 powerful questions that will give you the keys to unlock deeper and more profound love so you don't have to keep searching (or suffering) in disconnected relationships."

—**NATALIE KUHN**, spiritual teacher and co-CEO of The Class

"When we pose a question to someone we love and listen deeply to their reply, we not only learn, we deepen our human bond with them. In this moving book, Topaz Adizes gives us the profound gift of questions that will transform our relationships, and our lives, forever."

—**JEFF WETZLER**, author of *Ask: Tap Into the Hidden Wisdom of People Around You for Unexpected Breakthroughs in Leadership and Life*

12 QUESTIONS FOR LOVE

A Guide to Intimate
Conversations and
Deeper Relationships

by Topaz Adizes
Founder of The Skin Deep
& creator of {THE AND}

SASQUATCH BOOKS
SEATTLE

Printed in the United States of America

SASQUATCH BOOKS with colophon is a registered trademark of Penguin Random House LLC

28 27 26 25 24   9 8 7 6 5 4 3 2 1

Editor: Jill Saginario
Production editor: Isabella Hardie
Designer: Tony Ong

Front cover photograph: © Little Studio1 / Adobe Stock
Back cover photograph: © Kamran / Adobe Stock

Library of Congress Cataloging-in-Publication Data
Names: Adizes, Topaz, author.
Title: 12 questions for love : a guide to intimate conversations and deeper relationships / by Topaz Adizes.
Other titles: Twelve questions for love
Description: Seattle, WA : Sasquatch Books, [2024] | Summary: "Ask better questions, strengthen empathic listening, and practice vulnerability in conversation through 12 questions tested and proven by The Skin Deep's Emmy Award-winning work, perfect for combatting disconnection within your intimate relationships"– Provided by publisher.
Identifiers: LCCN 2023015953 (print) | LCCN 2023015954 (ebook) | ISBN 9781632174901 (hardcover) | ISBN 9781632174918 (ebook)
Subjects: LCSH: Love. | Interpersonal relations–Psychological aspects.
Classification: LCC BF575.L8 A275 2024 (print) | LCC BF575.L8 (ebook) | DDC 152.4/1–dc23/eng/20230622
LC record available at https://lccn.loc.gov/2023015953
LC ebook record available at https://lccn.loc.gov/2023015954

ISBN: 978-1-63217-490-1

Sasquatch Books
1325 Fourth Avenue, Suite 1025
Seattle, WA 98101

SasquatchBooks.com

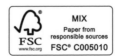

MIX
Paper from
responsible sources
FSC® C005010
FSC
www.fsc.org

For
  My Mother Tzia, who taught me integrity
  My father Ichak, who taught me passion
  My stepmother Nurit, who taught me art
      My wife Icari, who taught me intimacy
  and my two children, Cosmos and Lylah Oceana,
     for the lessons I have yet to
                   Learn.

CONTENTS

II. The 12

I. The Tools

III. Before You Begin

FOREWORD

One summer night in 2018, my sister, aunt, and I saddled into the booth of a sleepy diner, the two women sitting across from their respective husbands. Each of us ordered some late-night breakfast items from the tattered menus the waitress slid across the table. We'd just concluded a night of dancing and were ready to satiate our post-midnight munchies when my sister Jeanne pulled out her phone and declared, "Let's play this question game!" She is notorious for asking us to play games that drop us into less-than-casual dialogue at awkward and oft-inappropriate times, but we were all too tired to resist. About three intense questions in, it occurred to me that I'd played this game before. "What is the name of this game?" I inquired in between questions. "I think it is called {The And}," she responded before moving on to the next probe.

I met Topaz in late 2017, both of us inductees in the inaugural cohort of a social impact fellowship in New Zealand. We were quickly kindred souls, two fledgling entrepreneurs bound by a desire to help humanity achieve more authentic intimacy through the process of inquiry. My focus for more than a decade has been on self-inquiry as means for accessing what I call radical self-love, i.e., our inherent sense of worth, value, and divinity. Topaz was leading us to deeper interpersonal intimacy through his digital media platform The Skin Deep and a unique set of questions called {The And}. We each understood that the key to a world of personal and social thriving was to get closer to ourselves and each other. Much of the malaise and misery experienced in the world is a function of profound disconnection. We fear knowing and being known and thus we don't ask what would shred our self and social illusions. We avoid the hard questions that would dislodge the stories of trauma, because healing is scary. We evade what would unearth the already fractured foundations of many of our relationships because we believe it will render us isolated and unloved. All this evading and avoiding only robs us of the fecund possibilities beyond the status quo of our existence. We shortchange the magic that is inevitable inside of true connection, settling instead for a facsimile of relationship, a façade of intimacy. I love that Topaz has always known there was something greater in each of us if we could start asking the real questions and telling the truth to each other. I knew that something greater was possible if we could start telling the truth to ourselves. *12 Questions for Love* is an offering of practice with Topaz Adizes as a skillful facilitator holding the container for our truths to emerge with one another. Don't we all deserve such tender guidance as we practice our ever-expanding bravery together? I certainly think so.

I don't recall what I ate at the diner that night, but I do remember telling my sister what I admired about her and listening to my uncle tell my aunt what he saw as her greatest gift to their relationship. I remember feeling connected to each of them from a more honest place than before we arrived at the restaurant. A series of questions my sappy sister pulled up on her phone opened a space for a deeper indwelling of love between us. The expansion of that space in our world is why this book is so necessary. May these questions crack you and your loved one open. May you never close again.

—**SONYA RENEE TAYLOR**, activist and author of the *New York Times*-bestseller *The Body Is Not an Apology: The Power of Radical Self-Love*

WELCOME

Have you ever found yourself in the presence of someone you love dearly and had nothing to say? The silence not indicative of your care for the other, nor of your desire to connect with them, and yet there were no words you could grasp to articulate the depth or quality of your connection to them? Or have you found yourself in the same looped pattern of conversation with someone you love? Feeling as though you were treading the same path repetitively and it was simply exhausting? Even worse, it was deteriorating your connection.

Have you found yourself so in love that you want to forge an even deeper connection but are unable to find the tools or the experiences to help you build the next, greater version of what you sense is possible?

Have you experienced the desire to connect on a deeper level but fear that becoming more vulnerable will push the other away? That in leaning into the heartier parts of a relationship, you risk losing it all?

Have you questioned the value of intimate relationships? Or what intimacy really means? What is it in essence? How does it affect one's life? How do you build it? How do you maintain it? And on a more rudimentary level, what's the payoff?

My first response to you is: Welcome.

It is not a mistake you are reading these words. However you came to this book, there was something in you craving a new way to experience love, connection, and intimacy. I hope you're ready to take a deep dive and be open to the transformational power of deeper relationships, because you are in the right place.

· · ·

For the last ten years through the Emmy Award–winning project {THE AND}, I have been studying and watching humans of all types, and in all kinds of relationships, simply talk. But there is more to it. I've crafted the space for powerful, cathartic conversations to occur. I've created the questions that spark those experiences for the participants. I've trained others to hold the space, write the questions, and ultimately create these powerful moments for people across the gender, social, economic, and cultural spectrums to connect in new and profound ways.

I have spent thousands of hours watching the video recordings of those people in these exchanges. And I've learned a lot. I've learned about the human condition and its craving for raw and real connections with other humans. I've learned that we all yearn for that connection whether or not we know it. I've learned how the power of questions can change your whole perspective and thus how you experience your life. I've learned how challenged we are as a culture to be vulnerable with one another and have come to understand the payoff when we do. I've learned what listening, really listening, looks like. I've learned that the heart is built to love, and yet has to traverse through rugged terrain to find another loving heart. And I've learned that every relationship has its own unique space between that, which if accessed can provide rich nutrients to fuel growth and elevate a relationship to deeper levels, reminding us of the beauty and meaning of what it means to be alive.

All of these lessons have changed me. Through them I've learned about my own life's journey, which has led me to this place.

I am going to share everything I've absorbed from witnessing over a thousand conversations, as well as the lessons from my own first-hand experiences. You will walk away with the tools you need to deepen your connections with those most important to you. As couples therapist and bestselling author Esther Perel put it, "The quality of our relationships determines the quality of our life."

But what determines the quality of our relationships? I'd argue that it's the conversations we share with our partners—the depth and connection we cultivate and discover as we speak to our loved ones within a shared space. So what determines the quality of those conversations? What allows them to offer us a space for exploration, discovery, and connectedness? The quality of the questions out of which they arise.

• • •

I am going to offer you 12 meaningful, powerfully constructed questions to ask and the tools to create the space in which to answer them, thereby fostering greater connection in your relationship.

So thank you. I am grateful you are here.

And now, I invite you to explore the space between.

INTRODUCTION:
Where This Journey Began

We spend most of our lives looking for answers. In Western society, that's what we're taught to do. In the world we live in, it's those of us who produce results that get rewarded. Our definition of greatness is indelibly tied to accomplishment rather than inquiry. But what would happen if we took the time to question what we—as a society or as individuals—want to accomplish in the first place? Think about the difference it would make if instead of asking *How can I make more money to leave a legacy for my family?* more people asked *How can I create a better world for my grandchildren to live in?* The answers that might arise from that second question could set our entire species on a different—and I'd argue, far more sustainable—trajectory. What would our world look like if we shifted our focus to the questions we ask first, and then let the answers to those more thoughtful questions blossom?

I've seen how the questions we ask are far more important than the answers we seek. After all, every answer is shaped by the question from which it springs. Therefore, asking insightful questions can only lead us to better, more helpful answers. Could rethinking the questions that we ask ourselves heal social issues, protect the environment, fix polarized politics, even save the world? I certainly think so. But creating more desirable questions for us to ask ourselves as a society isn't something I have experience with. At least not yet. My expertise lies in asking powerful questions to create deeper connection, rediscover exploration, reinforce the sense of one's humanity, reinvigorate deteriorating relationships, and, I dare say, help heal pain. So, although I may not know for sure if shifting our focus to questions instead of answers will save the world, what I do know beyond a shadow of doubt from years of direct experience is that asking better questions can both lead us to a deeper understanding of intimacy and create a new, more vital path to journey upon.

• • •

My own journey through life has been defined by a search for intimacy. And that quest began some four decades ago with a question. I was four years old, playing with my younger brother. We were at my father's home and my mother was coming over to pick us up for some holiday dinner. By this point, my brother and I were well accustomed to our parents' divorce intruding on our lives. We were often shuttled back and forth between homes, with visits to court-delegated therapists in between as the judge evaluated the best custody schedule for us. To say that it was a messy divorce would be accurate.

My father came into the room where we were playing with our toys, looking distraught. He said that our mom would arrive soon to pick us up but that he wanted to be with us for the holiday and didn't know what to do. Wanting to help, I suggested that he write up a contract. It would stipulate that if she got us for this holiday, he would get us for the next one.

"Good idea," my father replied. "And what exactly should the contract say?"

Now, why would my father bring this up with his kids or put the onus of writing this contract on me? Who knows. But regardless, I, a four-year-old, proceeded to dictate to him roughly what this "contract" would say. Soon after, I heard the crush of gravel as my mom's big yellow Oldsmobile station wagon—a classic relic from the early eighties—pulled into the driveway.

I remember vividly how the lights of the car hung suspended in that heavy mist. When she got out of the car, emotional chaos ensued. I remember my father holding out the contract I'd dictated to him for my mother to sign. My mother flatly refusing as she grabbed my sobbing three-year-old brother and placed him in the car seat. Then, as she went to grab me, my father taking my brother out of the car seat and placing him on the doorstep to his house. I don't know how many times we were stuffed into and then yanked out of the car by our parents. I remember the feeling of hot tears streaming down my face as I begged my mom to sign the contract, not necessarily because I cared where we would be on what holiday, but just to end this painful hell of fighting.

My mother finally managed to get both my brother and me in the car and then pulled out of the driveway. Through the entire episode, she hadn't shed a tear. Staunchly aggressive but not emotionally vulnerable. She was very strong.

And then it happened. We'd come to a red light and were waiting for it to change. My brother's sobs had transitioned to whimpers. The warm tears had dried on my face. But while waiting at that light, I heard my mother begin to sob quietly. And that moment is when the first big question I can remember facing appeared in my mind.

Even at that age something about the delay in my mother's emotion, about the whole crazy situation from the moment my dad asked me to play mediator, seemed deeply and utterly off. Something was wrong in their relationship. Something was missing. I'll never forget sitting in the car and asking myself, *What is it? What is wrong here?* I couldn't know it at the time, but this moment marked the beginning of my quest to understand intimacy.

Finding My Bridge

Looking back now, it's clear that this was what was missing between my parents: real intimacy—the trust that's born of it, the willingness to be vulnerable that it affords, the powerful connection it facilitates. But I didn't know that at age four. Having never had it modeled for me, I didn't even know what real intimacy looked like. All I'd seen was that conflict between partners only ever ended in awful situations like the one my brother and I had found ourselves in that misty night. My parents' example had taught me that facing conflict head-on with a partner was so scary and undesirable that it'd be safer to have a child dictate a formal contract for both parties to sign than to have an honest and vulnerable conversation to work through it.

When I started dating and trying to create intimate relationships of my own, I found that my parents had unintentionally passed their aversion to facing conflict on to me. At the first sign of an issue with one of my partners, I'd protect myself from the emotional chaos I was certain was in store for us by asking myself *How is this going to end?* I'd only ever seen conflict devolve into yelling, pain, and an impasse through which nothing positive ever flowed. Therefore, to me, if there was any conflict, the ending wasn't in doubt; it was coming and it wasn't going to be pretty. Knowing what I know now, I can see how the question *How is this going to end?* didn't have many positive or constructive answers. But thanks to my limited understanding at the time of both how to create intimate connections and how to build useful questions, as soon as some conflict appeared, I'd ask it, and I'd get the only possible answer my past experience allowed: *This is going to end badly.* So I'd break up with my partners. At the first sight of conflict, I was gone. That was how I'd protect myself from more emotional pain.

It's no wonder I repeated that pattern over and over again. As we'll see in this book, leaning into emotional conflict can be one of the most fruitful ways to learn. Making friends with our conflicts and asking them what they have to offer us is how we break unhelpful patterns and move on to a greater, deeper understanding of our world, ourselves, and our relationships. But I hadn't realized that yet. Having lacked a model for intimacy in my childhood and having fled from any hints of it in my twenties, I lacked the sort of intrapersonal connections that would eventually offer me this valuable lesson. But looking back, I can see that the question *How is this going to end?* was another important signpost on my journey toward understanding how to foster deep connections. Sometimes you have to learn what not to do in order to find your path.

As I got older, the absence of intimacy in my life weighed heavily on my shoulders. I wasn't exactly conscious that it was intimacy specifically that was missing from my life, but I felt this powerful pull to seek *something* to fill the void in me with a thing I couldn't name but knew I lacked. When I graduated college, I looked around at my life and realized, nameless void notwithstanding, that I was supremely lucky. My parents were healthy. I had no student debt. My dad's job offered me a financial safety net, as I could always work for him. In a lot of ways, I was as free as a young person could be. And as all my friends were going to work at big consulting firms, which seemed to be the thing to do at the time, I wondered instead: *How can I spend my freedom—the most valuable currency there is—to serve my greater community?* No answer appeared right away. But I didn't need one to; I simply allowed that question to guide me.

With that important inquiry etched in my mind and heart, I took stock of what I knew about myself: I knew I didn't want to waste my life, I knew I was searching for something important (even if I didn't know what it was), and I knew that there was something about the magic of a video camera that excited me, that created an emotional response in my heart I felt called to follow. Somehow, I intuitively felt that the camera was the tool I'd need to find whatever it was I sought. And so, armed with little more than those few "knowns" and a video camera, in December of 1999 I set out into the world with a one-way ticket to Australia. I wasn't sure what it was I wanted to film exactly, but something about candid, honest exchanges between people drew me in. I traveled from Australia to Sweden to India, talking to people from all different backgrounds and filming those conversations. And it was during this period of what had initially seemed like aimless wanderings that I noticed something important.

The video camera I carried with me acted like a bridge into other people's worlds. It was a key that unlocked the doors they put up around their private lives. If you show up with a camera to film a documentary, people will share things with you they wouldn't normally share. Suddenly I was witnessing all sorts of intimate connections between people that I'd only just met and wouldn't have had access to otherwise. I was fascinated. Filming conversations like this was so captivating for me that I began to realize that this was what I'd been searching for: intimacy and connection. From my privileged vantage point behind the camera, I saw people build beautiful bonds with just a word. I saw couples gift each other verses of eloquent love poetry via a single, silent glance. I saw some human beings really communicate, truly relating to each other by paying full attention to their exchanges. And I watched as others completely ignored the needs of their fellow person or romantic partner, speaking for hours without hearing a thing the other said.

By becoming a filmmaker I had found what I'd been looking for, and upon finding it, I realized it was more precious than I could have ever imagined. More and more, as I became mesmerized by human behavior and connection, I began to realize that in our modernizing world this was something we were in danger of becoming less and less aware of, if not losing altogether. Having spent years honing my craft as a filmmaker, I sensed that this was the subject on which I wanted to bring those skills to bear. I'd found the answer to my question.

How can I make the most of my privilege and opportunity to serve my community, however big or small that community is?

I needed to document the invisible bond that forms between human beings, which we call intimacy.

But how?

Letting questions lead me down my path in life had gotten me this far. I wasn't about to stop following them wherever they'd take me next. I allowed my mind to fill with questions about how to best bring intimate connections into focus, both for the sake of healing my own wounds and as a way to give the world an offering of some value.

Illuminating the Space Between

Take a moment and ask yourself: *What is intimacy?* How do you experience it? Can you compare it across various relationships? Does it shift and change with different people, and what about in different cultures, languages, and communities? What is intimacy, really?

These questions feel difficult to answer definitively, even though plenty of theories abound. But one thing is for sure. We can't learn much about intimacy in a vacuum.

If you've never had a close relationship with another person, and especially if you've never examined one of those relationships with conscious awareness, intimacy may be difficult to assess. The key seems to be the strength of the connection you make and the willingness to open yourself to that connection that you bring to any interaction. The result, in my opinion, is that in a moment of intimacy your sense of humanity, or what connects us all, is heightened. Think about that moment when you looked in your lover's eyes and felt something so profound that you couldn't put it into words. Or that time you had an epic conversation with a passing stranger that gave you a sense of how incredibly beautiful and random life can be.

Intimacy is an invisible force, and personally that force gives me a greater sense of what it means to be human. When I travel from city to city giving talks, I always bring a pair of magnets with me. During my presentation, I'll bring them out to illustrate the unquestionable power and the illusive nature of the space between. When you hold two magnets close to each other, you can feel an energy between them. It's undeniably there; you can feel the push or the pull, but you can't see it. Much like there is a force between the magnets, there is also a force that lies between you and everyone else. The connection that forms between us that we call intimacy is no different. It exists in the space between. So imagine if you could sprinkle baby powder between those two magnets and then see those rays of connections stretching between them. That's what I wanted to do: bring that energetic connection into focus, making what is felt visible—in essence, illuminating the space between.

To accomplish this, I decided to use the tool that had served me so well thus far on my journey—the video camera—to film a simple conversation and see if that space between would reveal itself. In each session, two participants would sit across from each other and ask questions that had been tailored to their relationship. I would have each participant ask roughly a dozen of these questions in a prescribed order to create a space for connection and to allow a cathartic conversation to bloom. Participants would be presented with questions that were a surprise to them both (the first time they read the questions aloud was the first time they were seeing them) and could embark on a conversation they wouldn't have had otherwise. We would film these sessions with three cameras—one wide shot and two close-ups, respectively. Thus, the audience would see the participant's faces straight on, side by side, as we would split the screen into two panels, showing each close-up simultaneously. So as a viewer you not only hear the words the participants are using, but also see a sensory connection of them reacting to each other. It is in this way that we revealed the space between.

We titled this project {THE AND} because a relationship isn't you or I, us or them. It is you and I, us and them. It is "the and" that connects us. It is "the and" that is the conjunction of you and I that creates us. It is "the and" that is the space between. By focusing our attention and our cameras on that space, we were able to capture a clearer picture of what intimacy looks like than I'd ever imagined. By showing both faces simultaneously, one gets a sense of the threads that bind the two participants. The bipanel (and sometimes triptych format when we would show the wide shot) illuminates the space between, conveying the underlying connection beyond the words. This is a unique experience if you think about it. How often do you get to see a direct close-up of both people's faces as they unpack and navigate through emotional terrain? Either you are seeing the profiles of another couple have an intimate conversation, or you yourself are a participant in the conversation, seeing only the other person's face. As a viewer of {THE AND} you get to see both people straight on simultaneously. This is not a normal human experience in everyday life, and in that way it reveals a unique perspective we can rarely experience elsewhere.

· · ·

This became the format of our documentary project {THE AND}, which garnered an Emmy Award for New Approaches to Documentary in 2015, plus numerous other awards. It spread like wildfire through the internet, garnering hundreds of millions of views, and even saw celebrities like Robert De Niro and Anne Hathaway partake. The project has featured nearly twelve hundred couples across the spectrum of race, gender, culture, sexual orientation, and age, from eleven countries and counting. In addition to the broad scope of relationships covered, we have also had some participants return for subsequent conversations numerous times over the past ten years. Thus, {THE AND} boasts not only the breadth of a wide range of participants but also depth, as you can see change over time in a relationship. In essence, we were and still are building an archive of human relationships for our time—a library of humanity reflected in the emotional experiences shared through conversation.

During some conversations we filmed, I witnessed incredible moments of intimacy and connection, ones that I'll never forget for as long as I live. And while sometimes there seemed to be nothing going on in the room, when we would rewatch the conversation with the participant's faces side by side, suddenly you could see some exchange of value. The words and energy may have felt flat in the room, but {THE AND}'s bipanel format revealed something more under the surface. Even if one participant passed on answering a question entirely, the faces reacting to each other spoke volumes about their relationship. And that proved incredibly intriguing for me and for our growing audience. {THE AND} was working; it was illuminating that elusive-yet-vital space between two interconnected human beings.

In our early days, you'd never know what would happen. We would spend a twelve-to-fourteen-hour day hosting eight or nine pairs. Each for an hour or longer. We would let them go on for as long as they wanted or needed. I remember having this out-of-body experience once while filming in Amsterdam. There I was in a large warehouse with four lights illuminating these two people sitting opposite each other and three cameras recording their every exchange. And from this removed perspective I thought, *This is really fucking weird and incredible!* It's like studying humans being . . . humans? Our team likes to say we are really good at allowing humans to be exactly that: human. I believe the library of conversations we have built thus far is a testament to that. Each conversation is a surprising revelation. Some would be incredible in the room and others would seem to fall flat. Either way, we knew there was something to learn from each and every conversation and that we could capture that lesson with our bipanel format.

I began to wonder what was happening here. Why was this working, and what could my team and I do to make it better? What was the difference between the deeply connected exchanges and those that never quite got to a place of emotional depth? And so I formulated the following question for myself: *What is it about the conversations in which these sacred moments reliably occur that creates the space for true intimacy?*

As usual, no answer came shooting out of the clouds like a lightning bolt to strike me with instant insight. But I just kept this question at the forefront of my consciousness as I continued filming conversations for {THE AND}.

Finding the Answer in a Question

And then it happened. I got my answer. I was filming a conversation between Rafa, a tall man with ever-present brown eyes, and Douglas, with a calm and gentle demeanor, who were both in their forties and had been married for four years. In response to an earlier question, I had heard Douglas mention his mom. I noticed something in his voice that seemed to hint at a complicated, perhaps painful emotional substrate beneath his words. I figured that maybe if I wrote Douglas a question asking Rafa to reflect on Douglas's relationship with his mother, it might create a connected space in which Rafa's perspective could help Douglas find healing.

I watched Douglas pick up the card on which I'd written the question, and immediately his eyes started welling up. Before Douglas had even spoken, Rafa reached his hand out and wiped his husband's tears away. Douglas read the question out loud. "What change in me could I make to improve my relationship with my mom?"

Immediately Rafa looked up at the ceiling. I could see him sitting there in his partner's pain. The source of that pain might have been Douglas's relationship with his mother, but because of the strength of their connection that pain was Rafa's too. It started to rise up within him. Suddenly, both men were sitting there in a moment of silence, each pair of their red and watery eyes a perfect mirror of their partner's. Nothing was said, but I could see the raw brilliance and honesty of their intimacy shining as bright as could be.

After letting that moment wash over them, Douglas broke the silence to quip, "They're not even charging for this counseling session." The couple burst into shared laughter, tears still fresh on their faces.

This was exactly the sort of moment I hoped all participants in {THE AND} would get to experience. And what had caused it? A question. And not just any question. I'd thought it through carefully before writing it down for Douglas. It hadn't allowed for a "yes" or "no" binary response. It had invited a constructive result, had carried in its wording the potential to actively change things for the better. When Rafa's laughter died down and he eventually answered, his response was one that only he could have offered Douglas. He wasn't simply offering his opinion as Rafa the individual; he was speaking from the version of himself that's inextricably connected to his partner. He was speaking from that space between—what I call "the and."

• • •

Reflecting on that moment, I realized for the first time the true power that every question we ask carries coiled inside of it. I saw how crafting a question in a certain way allowed that power to spring out, creating a bridge that two people engaging in shared vulnerability could walk across to reach a beautiful, intimate moment. And just like that, {THE AND} was really off and running.

Over time, my team and I became experts at asking these kinds of powerful questions. We learned how to place questions in a certain sequence so that they were well-timed, built upon a solid foundation of trust and openness that had been established by previous questions so that they could reliably result in a deepening connection and illuminate "the and" between two participants. In my years of facilitating conversations like this, I can't say I've seen it all, but I've seen a lot. I've seen patterns. I've seen how our aversion to vulnerability and pain is compounded by a society that has its own stigmas of what is acceptable and what is not. I've seen the heart's natural impulse to love push through that maze of rules and fears time and time again in an effort to find and connect with another yearning heart, to feel for a moment, or for a lifetime, that it is not alone. I've seen how challenging it can be to put words to emotions, to actually articulate and impart one's depth of feelings to another. And I've seen the power that comes when that emotional articulation is successfully transmitted.

I've also seen how every relationship has a story out of which compelling, deep, and profound truths manifest. Take my parents, for example. After years of studying relationships by filming {THE AND}, I can see that despite their dysfunctional relationship, my parents were perfect foils to each other. From my perspective, my father's greatest fear was to be directly, intimately loved by someone. As for my mother, her greatest fear was to love directly, to intimately express her love to someone. In a way, they'd each found the perfect partner, in that their greatest fears were complementary and equivocal in weight and risk. The next step for their growth was equally scary for each of them. And yet the opportunity for both of them to face their fears through the other was presented by their union. Intimacy was equally risky and challenging for them.

Although they did not take that mutual leap toward developing deep intimacy, I can't help but marvel at the beautiful design I see in their relationship. Accepting intimacy and stepping into vulnerability could only have been accomplished through engagement with the other. It is from their relationship that I take away the belief that we find partners who uniquely offer us opportunities to grow and evolve as human beings. These opportunities are equally scary and challenging for both parties. But if we hold on to each other—with respect and trust and the mutual understanding that facing our individual fears together is the only way that we can jump together—and instead of falling, we can soar.

These are the kind of truths and perspectives that my experience with {THE AND} gifted me. But they're there for all of us to learn. You just have to ask the quality questions to access them. And that is one thing my team and I have become experts at: asking quality questions in a certain order to bring the sacred intimacy between partners into the light.

{THE AND} became my life's work, growing into a compendium of intimate conversations that I put up on the internet in the hope that by watching them people would become inspired to ask better questions and deepen their own connections. Shortly after launching {THE AND} documentary project, our audience kept watching these incredible exchanges and wanted to have them in their own lives. Thus I distilled questions from {THE AND} into a deck of 199 questions and created {THE AND} Card Game, and subsequently a digital version of the card game as an app. They are an easy way for people to experience meaningful, guided connections for themselves and bring the kind of questions my team and I created for participants into their own homes.

I knew that the information we were gathering from facilitating and watching the conversations that took place in {THE AND} was valuable. And I always felt that maybe one day, maybe around our ten-year anniversary, after having accrued a decade of experience and understanding, I would publish a book sharing all that I learned over the course of witnessing countless intimate and vulnerable conversations and on my own journey down the path of questions. It is my sincere hope that my experiences prove helpful to you.

However, I feel that this book's second offering is even more important. It lies in what can happen when you turn the information in this book into experiences of your own and have the sort of conversations I've witnessed in {THE AND} for yourself. Despite everything I've learned studying intimacy via my filmmaking, I do not have all the answers. I am not a scientist. I am not a guru. And I am certainly not a licensed therapist. I can only speak from my observations and experiences, which, although extensive, are subjectively mine. Hopefully by engaging in the conversation this book will guide you through and putting the tools outlined in the following pages into practice, you will get to make your own observations about intimacy, learn your own lessons about relationships, and deepen your understanding of what it means to live as a human being on your own terms.

The conversations from {THE AND} that I will draw on as case studies to illustrate why I feel each of the questions I've included in this book are so effective have all been edited in the cutting room, and thus reflect the unconscious biases of myself and my team. But the conversations that you will have outside of these pages will be experienced in their entirety, interpreted and processed by you and your partner and no one else. That is the offering I most hope you receive from this book: let it teach you to become your own teacher.

The Dalai Lama says that love is not a feeling. It is a practice. Stepping into "the and," into the space between, is an endeavor that enables you to practice love. Doing so gives you agency in deepening the quality of your life and the love in it.

How to Engage with This Book

Part I of this book focuses on tools to create the space for connection and intimacy. They help build the context in which an exchange can truly offer catharsis for growth.

Part II is comprised of the 12 questions that I've seen consistently deepen the connection between romantic partners. However, you can use these questions in any of your relationships where you have a deep sense of connection, not just your romantic relationships.

Part III offers advice on troubleshooting conflict that could arise during your conversation.

The intention is for you to read through the book and then have an intimate conversation of your own. To play, refer back to the 12 questions in Part II, which are listed starting on page 201, and ask each other these questions. Alternatively, you could read Part I and Part III, then play the question game with your partner by asking each other the 12 questions to have your own {THE AND} experience. After you play, read through Part II to understand why the questions created the experience and catalyzed so much between the two of you.

How to Play {THE AND}

Once you have finished reading and are ready to enter into a conversation with the clear intention of having a valuable, creative, and honest interaction, here are the guidelines I suggest you put in place:

- This conversation works best if the 12 questions are asked in the order they appear in this book. The reasoning for this is explained in depth later.
- Begin by looking each other in the eye for thirty seconds. Get grounded to the space and to each other. (Noting, however, that not all folks feel comfortable with eye contact. Please do what works for you—an alternative I suggest is simply breathing in tandem with your partner.)
- Each partner will have the opportunity to ask and answer each question, if they chose to, and the initial question-asker alternates from question to question. For example, if you ask your partner Question 1, once they have responded they will have the opportunity to ask you Question 1. Feel free to discuss each person's answer until you reach a natural conclusion (it is a conversation, not a test.). Once both of you have responded, move on to the next question, alternating who asks the question first.
- Try not to cut each other off. Wait until your partner has finished a thought before responding.
- You don't have to answer every question. This is very important. Maintaining the right to pass keeps one from feeling cornered. You earn the right to pass by looking the question-asker in the eyes for ten seconds and saying "pass." (Again, if you feel more comfortable breathing together, that's OK too.)
- Remember to have fun. Look at this conversation as a game you and your partner are playing with each other. If things get heavy or heated, you can refer to the Tools and the Troubleshooting sections for ways to defuse tension that might arise.

Those are the basic rules of {THE AND} game. Others that are helpful to make sure the conversation goes safely and smoothly if things get heated are: neither of you will raise your voice; no one will walk out of the room until the conversation is finished; and if the conversation needs to be cut short for any reason, you will skip to the final two questions and ask and answer them in order to close the space on a connective and healing note. We'll go over these guidelines in more depth later in Part III, where we review troubleshooting conflict.

At the end of the book I have included the video links to all the references I make to {THE AND} conversations so that you can see and hear them for yourself (page 205). I also share some alternate questions that I feel fit thematically at the same emotional beat of the conversation as the question you are exploring (page 201). They could be great to use the second or third time you sit down with your partner to have the kind of intimate conversation you are about to be guided through. Lastly, throughout the book I have placed some quotes that have come out of the library of {THE AND} conversations that have inspired me and hopefully will do the same for you. The links to the conversations in which these statements occur are also included.

Rather than treat this guided conversation as the pinnacle of your exploration of intimate conversations, I encourage you to look at it as a learning experience—a practice round for every profound conversation that you will have for the rest of your life. Think of it as the beginning of your journey down your very own path of questions. Who can say where it will lead you?

I: The Tools

In this section, you'll find the tools to create the space for connection and intimacy. They help build the context in which a conversation that truly gets to the heart of what is special between two people can thrive. Read this section before you start your own intimate conversation, with the 12 questions in Part II (page 55) as a guide.

STOP LOOKING FOR ANSWERS. CREATE BETTER QUESTIONS.

When was the last time you consciously asked yourself a question?

Take a moment and think back to the first thoughts that entered your mind when you woke up this morning. Play back your inner monologue and take a close look at the way in which your inner voice spoke to you in those first few moments of awareness. Chances are, it said things like, *I'm hungry. I think I'll have eggs for breakfast today. I better get moving so I'm not late for work.* At face value, these are all statements. But where did those statements come from? Why did you have those thoughts in the first place? They didn't just come from nowhere. Something inspired them. Something created a space that those statements needed to fill.

Try to go back to the moment just before you became conscious of those thoughts. What were they a response to? You probably weren't aware of it, but before your inner voice had the chance to speak up, a deeper part of you was silently asking, *How do I feel? What would I like to eat? What time is it, and how can I make sure I fulfill my responsibilities?* Your thoughts were all answers to questions.

The truth is, we are constantly asking questions—of ourselves, of each other, and of the world around us. But that's not the way that most of us experience life. Much of the time, the questions we ask elude our conscious awareness because we're only paying attention to the statements, the answers. This is no accident. The society we live in is obsessed with answers. Our culture has programmed us so completely to focus on them that often we can't hear the questions we ask ourselves. And even when we do hear them, how thoughtful are we about the kinds of questions we're asking? Or the way they're worded and the kinds of answers they are designed to elicit? Solutions, results, outcomes, and actions are valued so highly that we hardly ever consider the thing that creates and shapes the conscious and unconscious spaces out of which they appear. Rarely do we place the same level of importance and intention on the questions from which we hope our precious answers will arise.

This is a missed opportunity. By chasing after answers in our search for solutions to all sorts of issues—in our personal lives, in our relationships, and even globally—we are looking in the wrong place. We're making a mad dash for the finish line without any understanding of the racecourse we're running. Just as the course dictates the shape of a race, it is the question that gives shape to its answer.

· · ·

After having observed thousands of conversations in {THE AND}, I've seen firsthand how questions not only shape answers, but have the power to nurture and support the connection between two human beings. Our society underestimates that power, but if you learn first to recognize it and then to wield it, you'll find yourself in possession of an extremely valuable tool for having better, deeper conversations. But the power of questions can do so much more than that. It is the key to empowering your experience of being alive. Learning how to create better questions will give you the ability to shape not just your conversations but your perspective of the world, which in turn will allow you to shape your reality.

So how does this work in practice? Take a moment and imagine yourself asking a child if they want to go to bed or not. It's getting late, so you interrupt their playtime and politely ask, "Do you want to start getting ready for bed?" Drawing on the extensive research I've conducted over the past several years of fatherhood, statistically speaking, 98.8 percent of the time the answer will be a definitive "no," usually wailed at high volume. But what happens if you change the question? What if you ask the same child, "Do you want to go to sleep on the bed or on the couch?" Suddenly, staying up past bedtime is no longer an option. The child's answer can only be "bed" or "couch." This is an extremely rudimentary example of the power of questions at work, but you can see how here the question has shaped the answer. And every question—even questions with much higher stakes than bedtime—hold that inherent power.

Allow me another example. A friend of mine and his three siblings were raised by their mother, who at the age of thirty-five was diagnosed with multiple sclerosis. At first, she fell into a deep depression, asking herself the question *Why me?* She spent days in bed as her four children, twelve years old and younger, were carrying the weight of this dire news and doing their best to support their mother. The family felt lost, as their future seemed to be a path of difficulty and pain ahead. One morning, the mother made a simple change to her question. She added one word. *Why not me?* This changed her entire perspective on the diagnosis. The answers to *Why me?* placed her in a state of depression and apathy. The answers to *Why not me?* put her in a position of empowerment and action: why couldn't she be the one strong enough to carry this pain? Our mind searches for answers. Let it work to your benefit by focusing it in a direction that is constructive for you. Put more energy and attention on the question than the answers you seek.

Long before I became consciously aware of how to wield it, I was a big believer in the power of questions. Every documentary I've ever made began with a question. Not an idea. Not a concept. A question. It was through refining that questioning process and asking them in a myriad of ways that answers began to take shape in the form of a film.

This was my process—question first, result second—and it served me well. But it wasn't until I began to write questions for {THE AND} that the true power of questions and how they can shape our reality really hit home.

When I first started filming the conversations that became {THE AND}, I remember being overcome with one emotion in particular: gratitude. My fledgling documentary project would have been nothing without the vulnerability and openness participants from all over the world brought to conversations that they were courageous enough to engage in fully and gracious enough to let me record. Faced with their willingness to share the most intimate parts of themselves, I felt a responsibility to make sure I was giving them the most cathartic experience possible, one that would reliably deepen their relationships. So I began to deliberate over how to craft questions for them to ask each other that would do just that. The experience of watching Rafa and Douglas's conversation was one such reference point for me, one in which I came face-to-face with the power of questions in action. But the next step for me was to learn just what it was that had made the question Douglas had asked his partner so impactful.

The more I analyzed the kinds of responses, emotions, and experiences that specific questions provoked, the more I learned that the precise wording and sequence of a question is paramount. Two questions that seem similar on the surface but are worded differently can lead to a completely different answer. For example, having partners ask each other, *Why do we fight so much?* generates a laundry list of grievances. Because of how the question is constructed, the only possible answers will be centered on conflict and nothing else. While a question like this might have created some salacious, click-bait content that would have gotten {THE AND} a lot more views on YouTube, that wasn't my goal. I wanted participants to have the opportunity to learn something new about their connection with each other, to give them a chance to explore new terrain that may have been overlooked in their daily lives. I wanted them to experience meaningful growth as a result of the conversation we were guiding them through. So I tweaked the question. It became *What is our greatest conflict and what is it teaching us?* Now, the idea that the conflict between them carries an inherent lesson is baked right into the question itself. Posed in this way, a complete answer can't be a list of the same old issues a couple fights about. It must offer an opportunity for growth that the pair can take if they so choose. The offering is there. The choice is theirs. By reconstructing the question, participants were given the chance to reframe their conflict. The possible answers to this question were transfigured from a list of complaints and a feeling of disempowerment into an opportunity for two people to see how something that had been a source of pain in their relationship could become a gift that might help them grow.

Asking better questions can do much more than just facilitate deeper and more constructive conversations. It can be the difference between confidently making a pivotal life-decision and being trapped by doubt. When my partner was pregnant with our first child several years ago, we found ourselves wrestling with the question, *Where do we want to live?* It was a question that felt so big, so daunting, and so important, it consumed us both. For five months we traveled searching for an answer. We visited Santa Fe and Taos in New Mexico; Boise, Idaho; Bend, Oregon; Seattle, Washington; and Boulder, Colorado. Regardless of where we went, no place seemed like it met all the criteria for where we wanted to settle down and raise our family. One city would seem like a nice place to raise a toddler, but were the high schools there good enough? Would it be economically viable long-term? Would it consistently inspire us? Was this specific landscape the one we wanted to gaze out on every day of our lives for years to come? With so many moving parts, *Where do we want to live?* is a huge, complicated question. Unsurprisingly, our search for an answer didn't yield much more than a spiraling hurricane of stress that spun us both in dizzying circles.

Luckily, by the time my partner became pregnant with our second child and we once again found ourselves considering a move, I'd spent a lot more time thinking about the power of questions. And so, this time around we decided to reframe the question we asked ourselves. Instead of *Where do we want to live?* our question became, *Where do we want to live until our new baby is six months old that will also support us in creating a nurturing and loving environment for our young children, while inspiring us to give more of ourselves to one another?* This was a much easier, albeit longer, question to answer. Although it might have grown in total word count, changing the wording of our question shrunk what we needed from our new home exponentially. Now it just had to be a safe, nurturing environment, one with lots of nature and a good sense of community. Suddenly we had a newfound appreciation for the place we found ourselves in already. It didn't matter if we'd want to move somewhere else someday. For the time being, we could answer our question confidently and happily make a decision we felt met all our needs, no stress-hurricane necessary.

While paying attention to the questions we ask each other can have a huge impact on the quality of our relationships, reframing the questions we ask ourselves can alter our entire perception of the world. The story of my friend's mother with multiple sclerosis is a prime example of that. Think about some of the difficult questions that have come up for you over the course of your life. Questions like, *What should I do with my life?* are hard to answer, but *What does my passion revolve around, and how can I develop that passion into a skill that will offer value to others?* is much more specific and easier to align with whatever your trajectory is in any given moment. By wording the question like this, you're seeing the world through a lens colored by your desire rather than through one that's designed to satisfy expectations of the typical life-path. *Why don't they like me?* isn't particularly constructive, but *Why do I think they don't like me and what's the gift I can take away from understanding that?* might lead you down a path of self-exploration and to a healthier understanding of how you view yourself.

Or how about a question many of us find ourselves asking when something bad happens: that is, *Why does this shit happen to me?* What would happen if we changed the question to *What is the lesson in this shit?* Or, even better, *How come I'm so lucky this shit happens to me?* And what if we took it to the next level with *How is this shit the fertilizer for who I'm becoming?* By simply changing the question, you've given yourself an opportunity to grow and to appreciate all that shit you've dealt with as a substrate for the kind of discovery and development that might catapult you into just the sort of life you've been seeking. Why not give yourself the opportunity to see that right off the bat by harnessing the power of the questions you ask yourself?

Instead of focusing on the end result—the answer to your question—paying more attention to the question itself allows a more empowering, constructive solution to appear. By shaping the question, you shape the answer, and by shaping the answer, you shape your reality. So stop searching for answers. Create better questions. Your relationship with yourself, with your partner, and with every aspect of the world around you will only become stronger, more intentional, and more empowered.

WHAT MAKES A GOOD QUESTION

How do you leverage the power of questions to reliably elicit meaningful, deep responses?

After years of creating questions for more than a thousand conversations and carefully observing the experiences that they produced, I identified five key components shared by the most effective questions participants asked each other in {THE AND}. These questions all had a connective point of view. Or, in other words, they were focused on the space between the question-asker and the respondent. They were nonbinary and open-ended, structured to elicit more than a simple "yes" or "no." They empowered a positive or constructive result rather than creating destructive conflict. They were unexpected, usually connecting two disparate ideas. Finally, they were phrased as an offering to the respondent, rather than as a directive or an accusation. Ask a question that honors all five of these elements, and the vibrant, beating heart of any issue will reveal itself.

Let's dive a little deeper into each of the principles that make a good question in order to see their value and how they work in practice.

It Should Have a Connective POV

A question that has a connective point of view is about the space between the participants—that invisible, magnetic, connective space I call "the and." It explores the unique relationship between two people, rather than asking either of them to speak from their subjective perspectives. For example, *What do you think about love?* isn't as strong of a question as *How do you think we think about love differently?* Do you see how the latter example elucidates the connection between partners, placing the respondent in the shoes of the question-asker and thereby inviting them to see things from a different perspective?

Furthermore, the perspective that the respondent is invited to take in order to answer might appear to be that of the question-asker. But it's not; it's actually the unique point of view of the connection between them, of the relationship itself. Yes, you are asking your partner to share what they think you think about love, but can their response ever encapsulate your exact thoughts, feelings, wording, mannerisms, and affect? Even if their answer resonates fully with what you think about love, or any topic for that matter, the very fact that they're the one offering that answer makes their response a union of your thoughts and theirs. They are seeing the world through two sets of eyes—yours and their own. That shared vision is the connective point of view. Superimposed on each other, your viewpoints create a perspective greater than the sum of its parts. This is the invisible fabric through which love is shared and nurtured.

Exploring any issue from this perspective ensures that your shared connection remains the focus of the conversation. Questions that don't have a connective POV can elicit long monologues in which one person speaks at length about their preferences, expounds on their personal theories of life, or generally just rambles on about themselves ad nauseum. This can't happen if a question has a connective POV because both you and your partner will be a part of any answer that arises, keeping both of you engaged in the conversation at all times. Asking your partner, "What is life teaching you?" is fine, but it's not nearly as interesting or valuable to either of you as asking, "What do you think life is teaching *me*?" You can easily think about what life is teaching you alone. The other person isn't really necessary. However, the latter question is asking for your partner's reflection on your feelings, necessitating their participation. Now you get to hear their perspective on your experience. This might offer a precious opportunity to learn something new about them or something about yourself you'd never realized, and it will certainly be an opportunity to better understand the connection between the two of you.

A great way to discern whether a question has a connective point of view or not is to ask yourself if the answer it provokes will be unique to the relationship, or, in other words, if the answer it elicits will be different depending on who you're asking. If the answer will vary depending on who is asking it, then the question does have a connective point of view. If the answer could easily be the same no matter who asks it, then it does not. Let's say your partner asks you, "What is your greatest fear?" and you answer, "Spiders." If your father or your boss or your friend asks you the same question, will your answer be any different? Does it have anything to do with your connection to them, or only to your own relationship with your greatest fear?

Questions like *What is your greatest fear?* are fine if you're just trying to get to know someone on a basic level, but they don't particularly have the power to deepen your relationship with anyone. Many popular books have been written offering a list of important questions to ask your partner, but few, if any, of these books or lists take the connective POV into account. Too many of their questions will provoke the same response regardless of who is asking them.

Some years back, a set of questions developed by psychologists Arthur and Elaine Aron, the 36 Questions that Lead to Love, went viral via the *New York Times* in a 2015 essay called "To Fall in Love with Anyone, Do This." I've taken a look at the questions, and only seven of them even vaguely speak to the connection between partners. The rest are questions in which one partner is asked to express their thoughts or feelings from their own perspective. For example, *What do you value most in a friendship?* And *What roles do love and affection play in your life?* Do you see how your response to those questions will be the same whether it's your partner, your mother, or your waiter who asks it? It's not that these aren't important questions to ask when you're first getting to know someone, but once you've developed a relationship with another person, isn't it more interesting to learn about your connection with them? About the dynamic space between the two of you?

Let's go back to our arachnophobia example for a moment and learn how to bring a connective point of view into the question *What is your greatest fear?* A stronger version of that question, one that has the power to deepen your relationship with your partner, would be *What do you think I'm most afraid of and why?* or *When you think about our future together, what concerns you the most?* Now, the answer can never be the same if you pose it to two different people. The focus has been brought back to the unique connection between you and whomever you're speaking with.

It Should Be Nonbinary and Open-Ended

Few words can staunch the flow of a good conversation more quickly than "yes" and "no." If followed by a thoughtful and personal explanation, sometimes "yes" and "no" answers can lead you to interesting places, but do the best conversations between partners focus on objective truths, on absolutes and binaries? Or are they about the subjective truths that lie within the heart? Aren't conversations that explore the shades of gray between binaries more interesting? Whether something is true or not doesn't teach you nearly as much about your partner as asking them *why* they feel a certain way about something, *what* it is they feel, or *how* those feelings manifest in them. Therefore, questions that are open-ended, that won't allow a "yes" or "no" to keep the conversation in shallow waters, are the stronger choice for inviting depth into your conversations.

"Yes" or "no" answers are also an easy way for a respondent to avoid having to truly open up and give voice to the nuances of how they view and experience their connection with their partner. Ask the question, *Do you love me?* and you'll receive a simple, one-dimensional answer. But if you ask, *Why do you love me?* or *How do you experience your feelings of love for me?* or *When does your love for me feel strongest and when does it feel weakest?* the answer you receive will be a complex exploration of your partner's emotional self. This is especially important for difficult questions. A "yes," a "no," or an "I guess so" can serve as a shield your partner might put up in order to hide from vulnerability and the deeper truth that lies beneath those responses. But a nonbinary question offers them the opportunity to explore further. Can you see how asking, *Do you think there are things about our connection that we could strengthen?* gives the option to shy away from vulnerability and discomfort by simply saying "no," while asking *What can we do to make our connection stronger?* creates an opportunity to lean into a constructive conversation?

It Is Stronger When It Empowers and Aims for a Constructive Result

Let's look at the question *What do we most misunderstand about each other?* How constructive could an answer to that question be? And how likely is it that this question will offer an opportunity for growth?

As constructed, *What do we most misunderstand about each other?* sets you up to respond by outlining points of disconnection but not necessarily to grow from them. The best-case scenario here would be that you are made aware of something your partner experiences as a misunderstanding, but that you didn't view it as such.

But what if you strengthen the question by asking *What do we most misunderstand about each other and what can we do about it?* or *What do we most misunderstand about each other and why do you think that is?* Think about what can happen then. By nature of the question's wording, the entire emotional tone of the response changes. Instead of two people struggling under the weight of misunderstanding, you have now framed yourselves as a team, planning how to face it together or already learning its teachings. The idea here is to shape the question in a way that puts yourselves in a position to be able to build together.

So, is a question laying the foundation for you to take off and explore something with your partner? Or is it setting you up for conflict that will disempower your connection? How is it making your relationship more communicative, empathetic, resilient, and capable of growth?

Let It Be Unexpected

Sometimes we find ourselves trapped in the same patterns—of thought, of behavior, of emotions. After living inside these patterns for long enough, they can start to feel like our reality. They become the boundaries within which we think our lives must play out. But this is a fallacy, and often a dangerous one. Living inside the boundaries we unconsciously create for ourselves and our relationships can close us off to the many lush possibilities life has to offer.

I've found that those possibilities tend to arrive in unexpected ways. After all, if we're expecting the pattern we're stuck in to continue, anything that breaks us out of it will seem unexpected, won't it? Making unexpected connections is a great way to train ourselves to stay open to new possibilities and perspectives, to welcome mental and emotional flexibility into our minds and our hearts. Doing so in conversation with others allows us to step outside of whatever rigid ways we've been viewing our relationships and allow new paths to open up for us. This can be done in two ways. One is to connect two ideas that don't often go together. Such as:

1   Connect two ideas that often don't go together.

- How does conflict make us better?
- What is your favorite memory from your worst relationship?
- What do you fear gaining?
- What does making money cost you?
- What's the biggest mistake you made that was your greatest gift?

The other is to place one person in another's shoes to force them to find an answer from the other's perspective. Here are a few:

2   Place one person in another's shoes to force them to find an answer from the other's perspective.

- What do you think I understand about life that you don't yet?
- What do you think is the hardest thing for me about being your friend?
- What do I misunderstand about you and why do you think that is?
- What do you think I think is my sexiest quality?
- What's a mistake you see me make repeatedly and why do you think I do it?

Do you see how all of these questions bring two unexpected ideas together, or place one person in another perspective, and in doing so invite the respondent to step into an unfamiliar perspective on a possibly familiar issue?

Time and time again, I've seen unexpected questions provoke cathartic emotional responses and meaningful revelations in participants in {THE AND}. Let's take one of my favorite conversations, which always manages to bring tears to my eyes, that we recorded in Wellington, Aotearoa (New Zealand), between John, early forties, bleached-blond, cropped hair, and his son Curtis, sixteen, with glasses, dressed in mostly black and with a heart-opening sincerity.

Curtis is neurodivergent and his family has always been very attentive to his needs. Knowing this, I wrote this question for John to ask his son: *What do you think is the hardest thing for me about being your father?* When John asked this question, the sense of relief he felt at finally having the opportunity to be seen in this way by his son was palpable. He let out a slow breath and his shoulders dropped as all the long-held tension seemed to escape. I wondered if John ever got to ask a question that placed Curtis in his shoes before. The space was created where John was seen by his son, possibly for the first time, in a different way than what their relationship had provided up until that point.

Connecting dots that we might have never thought to connect creates a new space to live in and makes a new connection in any relationship, thus opening up new ways of being together.

It Is Most Effective When It's a Gift without Judgment or an Agenda

There is a key distinction to be made between pointed questions that demand an answer and those that are presented as an offering, a gift. An offering is an invitation to explore something new or to impart a rarely expressed opinion. Conversely, questions that seek to extract an objective fact might be experienced as manipulative, have ulterior motives, and make a respondent feel boxed in. Can you feel the difference between the questions *When was the time I disappointed you most?* and *When was a time you felt most disappointed by me?* It's subtle, but it can make all the difference in the way your partner feels as they respond and in the response itself. The latter question is asking about *a* time versus *the* time, therefore allowing for flexibility, versus demanding something specific. Furthermore, it's asking when the respondent *felt* the most hurt versus a time they were objectively hurt. That tweak makes it personal to the respondent's experience and notes it as such. Rather than placing the question-asker in a position to be the arbiter of the truth, deciding if they did indeed disappoint their partner or not, it allows them to recognize the validity of their partner's subjective experience.

Let's look at another example. Which question would you rather answer: *What is the most painful thing you've done in our relationship?* or *What do you believe is the most painful thing you've done in our relationship?* Note how by adding the words *do you believe,* the second option softens the language so the question becomes about your opinion of a possibly painful action, rather than requiring you to admit definitively that you have done something that caused your partner pain. The question has been turned into an offering for you to discuss an event, instead of forcing you to try to make a claim about what you think is objectively true. This way no one is being set up to be attacked. It's much easier and safer to say to your partner, "This is my experience" versus "This is the reality."

It's true that not all interpersonal behaviors in a relationship are subjective; some just are objectively hurtful. I'm not proposing here that everything that happens in a relationship is up for interpretation. However, after years of honing how I write questions for {THE AND}, I've found that the best conversations come when questions are posed as opportunities for inquiry, which participants can choose to step into or not. It's much easier to shake an open hand than one that's pointing a finger at you. I've found that if the questions written for participants are too pointed, if they push you or your partner too hard to have a certain experience, the natural response will be for either of you to push back and possibly close off to the other. That's the opposite of what you're looking for if you're trying to honestly explore your connection in the space we hope to create.

HOW TO CREATE A SAFE SPACE TO HAVE CONVERSATIONS

Quality conversations can only take place when both partners feel they are in an emotionally safe space. Period. If either of you feels unsafe, even a perfectly constructed question won't be able to pry open the defenses you'll have instinctively raised around your heart. But be wary of conflating safety and comfort. They are not the same, and there is a key distinction to be made between the two. Safety is to be cultivated and maintained at all times, filling the space with a mutual understanding of shared intention, motivation, care, and clear guidelines. Comfort—emotional comfort—on the other hand, is something that I'd invite you to let go of as much as possible as you enter into your intimate conversations.

Discomfort is a necessary prerequisite for growth. How can any of us expect to experience the novelty that allows for positive change while locked inside the plush and familiar prison of our comfort zones? Feeling safe enough to explore your vulnerabilities together is paramount, a critical prerequisite for stepping into the conversation this book will guide you through. Understanding why you are having this conversation, the intention behind it, and what the rules are creates an emotionally safe space in which you can transmit your ideas vulnerably and in such a way that hopefully they can be received by the other.

• • •

Why do we go to the theater to see a movie or a play? We do it because we know we are in a safe space in which to feel the sadness or fear or heartbreak or anger we see a character experiencing. Meaning we are clear on the shared intention of the space, the motivation of being there, the care that is allotted to everyone, and there are clear guardrails to the experience. We have entered the theater with the intention of having that kind of experience. What's more, we have permission to watch these characters in their most intimate moments. We also know that the stage is where the actors perform, the seats are where we, the audience, will witness it, and that the boundary will not be crossed. It is both a safe space for us to experience intense feelings and to step into the role of the voyeur.

Now think about watching two people fight on the street. That's a very different experience from observing two actors fight on the stage. Part of you might naturally want to watch the street fight unfold; after all, it is a tantalizing expression of powerful human emotion. But at the same time, you feel pangs of guilt at invading the private space of others and waves of discomfort as your own space gets invaded by feelings and emotions you may not feel safe enough to sit with having gone out into the world with the sole intention of buying some groceries.

So, what's the difference between these two scenarios?

Framing, Context, and Permission

Imagine if your partner were to walk up to you as you're reading this book and suddenly ask, "Why do you love me?" completely out of the blue, without setting up a space or entering that space with a clear shared intention. What would your reaction be? Would you calmly drop into your feelings and begin to explore the multifaceted beauty of your love for them? Doubtful. Instead of thinking about why you love them, you'd be wondering, *Where is this coming from? What did*

I do? Did I leave the toilet seat up again? What do they want from me? Do they think I'm having an affair? The point is, you wouldn't be focused on answering the question they asked; instead, you'd be focused on trying to construct a context out of which a question of that magnitude might logically arise.

Just like a play or a movie creates a framing in which certain things are permissible to witness and experience that might not be in daily life, before having a deep conversation with your partner, it's important to frame what you're doing and to enter into this experience with the shared intention for this kind of cathartic and honest conversation to unfold, bound by rules that will keep you both safe.

That's why it's important for both participants to understand that they are willingly and intentionally entering into a space created specifically for conversations like this to happen. Using the 12 questions in this book (or any of {THE AND} card decks if you want more questions) to guide your intimate conversations can be helpful because they automatically and immediately frame your conversation as a game. By deciding to play that game, you've brought the intention of answering connective questions with you into the experience. But when you aren't using the cards, contextualizing the experience as something that has different rules than daily life is key for a conversation to be successful. Call it a game if you like. In fact, I'd encourage you to frame the conversation with as light and playful language as possible. Remember, while this conversation could lead you into levels of vulnerability and discomfort that allow you, your partner, and your relationship to grow stronger and wiser, it could also be an experience filled with laughter and pure unadulterated fun. Laughter can be a powerful teacher, one that we often underestimate. Referring to this conversation as a game will both lighten the atmosphere of the space you're creating and reinforce the idea that, as with every game, there are rules built into the experience you're about to step into.

Rules and Boundaries

Rules are not a bad thing. They are a tool in and of themselves. Ask any artist and they'll tell you that creative limitations—the boundaries or rules within which they create their work—are what allow them to thrive and make their best art. A painter who hasn't first given herself the rule that she will paint on a canvas or on a specific wall would be totally lost when determining the dimensions, scale, and perspective of her work. If I were to make a documentary without the rule in mind that it can't exceed a length of two hours, I might spend years struggling to create a ten-hour monstrosity that no one would be able to sit through. Similarly, rules that give boundaries to a conversation give shape to its space and scope, ensuring the requisite safety for participants to allow themselves to be vulnerable.

One of the main reasons many couples feel more comfortable discussing their issues in front of a therapist is because a therapist's office is a space governed by rules and mediated by a referee. Couples therapy can be an important and useful tool. It's one that I've used myself and have found effective. When undertaking your own conversations outside of couples therapy, you can be mindful in creating your own space and rules, so you can learn the skills needed to become your own referee. The two of you will have created an environment of safety that encourages honesty, openness, and self-discovery all on your own. Just sitting in the power of having accomplished that together can be huge for building trust in each other. Without anything actually "happening" or being "achieved," sometimes just being in a nurturing space you've created can be enough.

Let Go of Any Agenda

Entering the conversation openly is very different than going in with an agenda or expectation. The intention to have an exploratory conversation about your relationship is an open one; it allows for all possibilities. But sitting down expecting that something will happen or, even worse, because you want to fix your partner or change them is setting yourself up to demand a certain result or behavior from your partner. If the idea is to explore fluid dynamics, unexpected perspectives, and new ways of being together, won't bounding your experience in specific expectations only restrict where this experience might take you? You can't learn something new if you're only playing with what you already know. The only objective of this experience is for you to be together, intimately connected in a safe space and honestly responding to the questions you invite into that space, allowing for you to discover things—about them, about yourself, and about your connection to them. Trust in yourself, in your partner, and in the experience itself that whatever comes out of it will be right, even if that's just laughter or confusion or not much at all. If you've set rules and created a space in which you both feel emotionally safe, it almost certainly will be exactly what's needed, no matter how uncomfortable the conversation gets.

The path of growth is lit by your fears. Leaning into them wherever they appear and facing them together in a space where you both feel safe enough to be vulnerable—but confident enough to sit in discomfort—will build trust, strengthen your connection, and develop your relationship beyond where it currently exists.

Physical Space

Now that rules, boundaries, and intentions have been established, it's important that you feel comfortable in the physical space. This way you won't be distracted and can fully step into emotional discomfort. When filming {THE AND}, my team and I came up with a few tricks to help facilitate this. We like having participants seated on chairs that don't squeak and on top of a comfortable carpet. We also place a candle somewhere in the room if only to have a sense of energy moving through the space. The point really is to make it feel cozy and unintimidating. Once participants sit down, we ask them to count from one to ten, raising their voice from whispering to yelling, before they begin their conversation. This way they feel like they auditorily own the space. Directors crouch down to talk to participants, so participants are allowed to speak from a position of power. They are spoken up to versus down to. The director also makes solid eye contact to help bring the person into the space and to model this behavior for them in hopes that they'll do the same in the conversation itself. These are some of the techniques for making participants feel like the unfamiliar space in which they are being filmed is theirs. If you're in a very familiar space, like your kitchen, you probably won't need to kick off your own deep conversations by yelling, "Ten!" But make sure you're cognizant of the space you're in. Are there loud sounds going on around that can distract you? Is there a lot of movement going on that will pull you away from the moment? And is this a space in which both you and your partner feel like you're on equal footing? Make sure you are somewhere that both of you feel equally comfortable and, if possible, are positioned so that you're at eye level.

That last point is extremely important. Maintaining eye contact during this experience can be even more powerful for enriching your connection with your partner than any of the words you'll speak. We always make sure to have participants take thirty seconds to just make eye contact before they ask their first question, because we've seen again and again just how potent this moment can be. No matter who we are, where we're from, or what we look like, all human beings have the same black onyx pupil. These shining gems that all of us carry are referred to as the windows to the soul for good reason. What indescribable beauty, what inarticulable truths have you seen swimming in the depths of a partner's eyes? Start your conversation by taking time to explore them. No matter what you find there, looking into each other's eyes will reinforce the commonality we all share and ignite the flame of emotional intimacy before either of you have even spoken a word.* The idea is to ground your body in the space to become as present as you can.

*If direct eye contact is not possible or too uncomfortable, I suggest facing each other, closing your eyes, and breathing in unison for thirty seconds.

DEEP LISTENING

Deep listening is an essential tool that will help you engage with your partner on a more profound level once your conversation is in motion. It is the ability to let your partner's words into your body and hear how they resonate within it. Deep listening allows you to really take someone in, which is the necessary foundation for any truly connected interaction. Before you learn to speak, you have to learn to listen.

At its most basic level, deep listening means *feeling to listen*—feeling yourself and what the other sparks within you with your entire presence. To engage in deep listening, you focus both your mind and your body on what your partner is expressing. You're not thinking about what you'll say next. In fact, when engaged in deep listening you aren't really thinking at all. Instead, the totality of your attention is given over to two things: the words your partner is saying and how those words make you feel in your body.

Now let's clarify what I mean by "feel" or "feelings." I do not mean your urges. I mean what you feel in your bones. There is a difference between your urges and your sense of truly knowing. *I really, really want to have that pizza* is an urge. *I really don't want to be around that person because they are so arrogant* is also an urge. We often confuse feelings with urges. I am not talking about surface-level feelings. I mean the times when you just intuitively know. It's listening to what your body is deeply feeling versus superficially reacting to.

Have you ever gone shopping, online or in a mall, and you're looking for something—a gift, or something for your home—and the first thing you see you just know is perfect? It just feels right. But you tell yourself that you should keep looking to see if there is something better or for a cheaper price. And you spend the next hour going to all the other shops only to return to the very first thing you saw. Or when you are somewhere in public and someone catches your eye for some reason. You don't know why but you have the feeling you should speak to them. And it's not coming from a place of desire or physical attraction; it's something else. You're not sure why, but you just sense that there is some reason for you to have an exchange with them. Often the rationale doesn't make sense, but there is a deep intuitive sense of knowing. Then you speak to them and there is some beautiful synchronicity or some useful information they provide you with that you've been searching for. Or in the case that you do not engage with them, you find yourself still thinking about them for the rest of the day for no justifiable rhyme or reason. That is the level of feeling that you drop into when you're engaged in what I call deep listening. Trusting this feeling that your body and heart are communicating to you, much like your intuition. It doesn't have to make sense. It has its own logic, which may not be understood by you now but will likely be revealed later.

So how do you do this? Well, it's similar to how you let your thoughts go when in meditation, dropping into your body and becoming aware of any feelings—physical and emotional—that arise as your partner speaks. Did your shoulders just tense up? Did what they just say make you feel anxious? Did their words send ripples of pride or longing or tenderness flowing through your stomach? Did the pause that followed their statement give you a sensation of cliff's-edge vertigo? By focusing only on what your partner is saying and how your body responds, you'll become so wholly present in the conversation that you will find yourself effortlessly connecting with both your partner and the highest form of your being.

• • •

Right about now, you might be asking, "How will I participate in a conversation to the best of my ability if I never get the chance to think through what I'm going to say? My brain does all the talking, not my body. How do I know what my body is saying?" This is a completely understandable concern. We're so used to relying on our minds rather than our bodies that we have little if any experience witnessing the potent wisdom our feelings carry. But trust me, it's there, alive and well in your emotions. Feelings and emotions are stored in the body. All you need to do to welcome it into the conversation is slow down and make space for your feelings to speak through your body. A great way to do that is to pay attention to your breath. Is it deep or shallow? Where does it go? Where does it not want to go? Where does it get stuck? These are indicators of where the tension exists in your body and can quickly ground you into deep listening.

In the modern era that can feel like a tall order. As our world becomes more and more suffused with technology, there's a near-universal impulse to speed up, for everything to be as efficient and on-demand as possible. In a present and a future so focused on *doing*, the slow, organic practice of *feeling* is in danger of being lost. At the very least, we've gotten rusty. But it's our human ability to feel and to be aware of our feelings that differentiates us from technology and guides us toward something more profound. No matter how advanced artificial intelligence becomes at thinking faster than any of us can even comprehend, it will never have the same capacity to feel as we do. It is an unalienable superpower that we all share.

Feelings also happen on their own time. They can't be rushed or sped up to supercomputer speeds. Therefore, once your partner has finished speaking and you have finished listening, both to their words and to how those words have made you feel, it's OK for there to be a beat of silence. In fact, I'd encourage you to take a moment to let that open, fertile space bloom. It's on that blank canvas of silence that you can begin formulating your response. And if you've been practicing deep listening, you probably won't have to think too hard about what it will be. Often, you'll find an insightful response waiting right there for you. You'll have been guided to it effortlessly by the intuition in your body. Allow yourself to articulate it even if it doesn't quite make sense. It's what your body is telling you. So express it and see where that leads. It may bring you to a place you couldn't get to otherwise if only reacting with your mind and your cognitively processed thoughts.

I first became aware of deep listening while working as a filmmaker. Whenever I'd set out to make a documentary, I'd find myself conducting hours and hours of interviews. As I asked my subjects question after question, I started to notice that the more attention I paid to how an interviewee's words were making me feel, the better my questions became. Whenever I'd try to get a step ahead of them and go on autopilot, smiling and nodding as they spoke while I wracked my brain for the next great question to ask, the questions that I'd come up with were usually disconnected and flat. They wouldn't elicit reactions and statements that were insightful but rather would receive generic responses—things one expected or that didn't carry much emotional weight. But if I really tuned into my subject, into myself, and into the connection forming between us, I'd become so fully present in the conversation that I could feel the question to ask next. It would intuitively come to me, effortlessly manifesting from just listening to my body. At first it was hard to trust that this would happen. It wasn't easy to let go of my mind's need to have the next question all queued up and waiting to be jammed into the first sliver of silence that appeared. But I saw time and time again that if I just dropped into my feelings and was really present with another person, the most appropriate question for that moment appeared. It happened so effortlessly and reliably that it almost felt like I was opening a portal to something or somewhere else. Call it the collective unconsciousness, the source, the universe, your higher self, or whatever makes most sense to you, but those perfect questions seemed to come from some other, wiser consciousness outside of myself.

Once I really began to trust that this process worked, I committed to it fully. I conducted interviews like this for years, but I never really considered giving the tool I'd stumbled upon a name until I started working on {THE AND}. I had observed such a vast number of conversations that I began to realize there was a danger in not practicing deep listening. I noticed that even when a participant was paying close attention to what their partner was saying, if they weren't tuned into their emotions they tended to respond with what I call a cultural mantra, or societal programming, rather than something that was true to this specific interaction or their specific relationship.

I remember filming a series of conversations between participants who were single and meeting for the first time to explore if there was a romantic spark between them. Whenever the question *Why do you think I'm still single?* was asked, a huge number of participants would quickly fire off the rote response: "Because you're still figuring yourself out." This happened so many times and in so many different conversations between so many completely different people from every background imaginable, I just couldn't buy that it was an organic response born of a participant connecting with their own unique truth. I felt like it had to be one of these cultural mantras—something that society programs us to think is the appropriate response in a given situation.

Is this even true in the first place? Is being alone really the best way for us to figure ourselves out as it pertains to how we relate to others? What better way to discover who you are than by observing yourself engaged in the dance of a relationship with someone else, learning from them and learning from your reactions to them? This is why it's important to bypass the mind and look to the body, where feelings reside, to foster deep and truthful connection.

Just as "the and" alludes to the space between two people, it also alludes to the space between the mind and the body. It is that connection between the body's feelings and the mind's ability to articulate those feelings where we can drop into deep listening. Connect to the body, listen for the feeling, and trust what it tells you.

Mechanics of deep listening

- Focus your conscious attention on what your partner is saying.
- Maintain a curious awareness of how you are feeling, physically and emotionally, from moment to moment.
- Don't try to look for your response until your partner has finished speaking.
- When they have finished, stay tapped into your feelings and perhaps the resonant response will be there waiting for you, even if that response is an embodied and connected silence. Remember, it doesn't have to make sense. Simply let the body speak.
- Paying attention to your breath is an excellent way to tune in and reconnect with your body.
- Trust your intuition and whatever comes up and then boldly share from that space.

If you only know one thing about the French philosopher René Descartes, it's probably that he shook the foundations of seventeenth-century thought by declaring, "I think, therefore I am." While this might have been revolutionary in his day, these days, in an era where the act of cognitive processing will increasingly become the work of computers, I believe that human beings—and especially human relationships—would benefit greatly from changing Descartes's famous adage to "I *feel* therefore I am." That's a motto that could revolutionize cognitive philosophy and the way science is shaped in the twenty-first century.

EMOTIONAL ARTICULATION

Should you step into a clearly outlined space and explore via deep listening the answers brought up by powerful, well-constructed questions, the result is that you will improve the practice of what I call emotional articulation. This is the practice of giving voice to our own emotions in such a way that their power and weight are felt by whomever is listening. You might have heard of the (now slightly outdated) term *emotional intelligence*, the skill of being able to read, understand, and empathize with both your own and other people's emotions. Emotional intelligence is important for having these conversations, but it's just the first step. Emotional articulation takes the skill of understanding emotions and brings it out of the abstract realm by putting words to those feelings.

Learning how to express your emotions in a way that's honest, articulate, and intelligible to your partner will take the depth of your conversations to another level. But doing so isn't as easy as it sounds. In our society it's rare for a person to grow up learning this skill. Many of us experience emotions differently and many of us struggle to put words to our emotions. Often when we try to do so, our culture frowns upon the heartfelt expression of our feelings, telling us that we're speaking in cliché or being "cheesy." Unlearning that conditioning is a process. It can make getting the hang of emotional articulation feel uncomfortable at first. But the act of having conversations like the ones outlined in this book is an opportunity to hone this skill. Every time you sit down with someone and have a connective conversation, you'll find it gets easier to put words to your feelings. Luckily, it isn't necessary to be a master of emotional articulation for these conversations to be successful. However, having these conversations will definitely improve your skill of emotional articulation.

I remember watching my brother-in-law play {THE AND} Card Game with his daughter one time. We were all sitting around a large table having just finished dinner. It was Christmastime and the fireplace was burning nice and warm. His two teen daughters really wanted to play the game, so we pulled out the family edition. My brother-in-law is a kind, generous man who cherishes his family above all else. But when he sat down to play the game that evening, he hadn't had a lot of practice articulating his emotions. As the conversation between all of us unfolded, at one point his nineteen-year-old daughter pulled a card with the question *What is something you appreciate most about me that I don't realize?* We all went around the table sharing our reflections to her. When it was her father's turn, I could see his expression change. Clearly, there were heavy emotions inside of him that wanted to get out and express themselves. But he couldn't find the words. He sputtered and stammered, but the harder he tried to express his feelings for his daughter, the more difficult it became for him to articulate them. A wave of emotion was hitting a dam, eventually slipping out of his tear ducts because he couldn't channel those feelings sufficiently into words.

The moment was extremely powerful nonetheless. Through their eye contact and their willingness to just sit there together in that space, the essence of the emotion was transferred from father to daughter. It just wasn't articulated. Regardless of what he said or didn't say, she could still feel her father's love. Wouldn't it have been a beautiful gift had he been able to put words to the emotions he was feeling? By experiencing that moment, my brother-in-law got the opportunity to practice emotional articulation, stretching his expressive muscles so that next time he'd be able to get that much closer to putting words to his sincere feelings.

So how do we learn how to do this in our own conversations? The best advice I can offer is that overcoming the natural discomfort many of us feel when expressing our emotional selves takes practice, practice, and more practice. Luckily, in deciding to have the conversation outlined within the following pages, you have already given yourself a golden opportunity to practice this skill. As you ask the 12 questions in this book or play {THE AND} Card Game, pay attention to the ease or difficulty with which you are able to translate the spectrum of feelings your conversations provoke into the medium of words. Brené Brown, the acclaimed research professor at the University of Houston and bestselling author, says in her incredibly helpful book, *Atlas of the Heart*, "Language is our portal to meaning-making, connection, healing, learning and self-awareness. Having access to the right words can open up entire universes." This is why the endeavor of her book is to map out some eighty-seven emotions with words. Having common understanding of what words connect to which emotions can make it easier to understand one another.

As you and your partner ask each other questions, make sure you remain in a place of deep listening as much as possible. Deep listening can be one of your greatest allies in strengthening your ability to articulate your emotions in a way that is honest and true to your unique perspective. Remember how in deep listening you tap into your body, paying attention to intuitive feelings that come up and allowing a response that's right for any given moment to appear? Following your feelings might have led you to an image, or to an anecdote from your life that at first seems unrelated to the question that was just asked of you. No matter how strange or tangential it might seem, try just running with it. Begin to speak it out no matter what it is. You can begin with "What comes up for me is . . ." or "When I feel that, I . . ." Trust that your intuition has guided you to exactly where you need to be. If you're someone who struggles with emotional articulation, this can be a powerful exercise in expressing your feelings in metaphor and story-telling—two of the most artful ways of wrangling things as expansive as emotions and stuffing them into those tiny little containers we call words.

In addition to listening deeply to yourself, don't forget to pay attention to how your partner's words make you feel. Perhaps you'll notice that they have a vibrant emotional vocabulary and you'll be able to welcome some of their methods of self-expression into your own process. Sometimes our partner can be a great model for the level of emotional articulation we aspire to, and the more you engage in these kinds of conversations with them, the more you will learn.

Another extremely valuable resource of people modeling effective emotional articulation is {THE AND} itself. I invite you to check out the hundreds of videos of conversations we have made available on YouTube. Watch them closely and see where you feel participants are excelling at or struggling with emotional articulation. A good place to start is with Ben and Sidra's videos. They are a married couple who have returned to {THE AND} many times throughout their relationship, and their skill at expressing their feelings is mesmerizing to watch.

One of their more recent conversations for {THE AND} begins with Sidra—a tall, striking woman whose brown bangs end just above matching brown eyes—asking Ben, "What have I done that surprised you most this year?" Ben takes a deep breath, aims his gray-green eyes up at the ceiling for a moment, and allows himself to drop into his feelings. They lead him to a powerful memory, which he shares in rich detail and with full emotional engagement.

"I was going through your backpack," he begins, and then bursts into laughter as he hurriedly adds, "because you asked me to get something!"

In Sidra's backpack, Ben found a mess he colorfully describes as a "ferret's nest." It was overflowing with the hastily stashed and long-forgotten detritus of Sidra's life, including "a completely rotted banana. It was like a month old; it wasn't like a week old." Ben allows for a moment of shared laughter between him and his partner before letting his emotional connection to the memory lead him back to a less playful, more serious state. His smile fades and a passionate intensity enters his eyes as he moves toward the heart of his story.

"At the same time, you were on the phone with the insurance agent, talking about the fire, and I was listening to you." In a flash, his entire body becomes animated with delight from head to toe. Beaming at Sidra, he continues, "It was watching these two seemingly unable-to-exist-at-the-same-time realities that were part of the same woman . . . It was watching you just execute, execute, execute—with a baby on your hip and all the other things that you have on your plate— and also being an incredible mother at the same time."

For me, Ben's body conveys his internal emotions to his partner just about as completely as humanly possible. The pure happiness he felt at watching his wife dance through an overwhelming situation with grace is visible in his gestures, movements, and in every smiling muscle of his face. The wonder he feels at Sidra's strength, juxtaposed with a backpack that clearly shows just how stressful and hectic life was for her in that moment, pours out of his eyes. The love he feels for both her competence and vulnerability and the elation he feels at getting to bear witness to both in the same moment is crystal clear.

Ben has shown both us and Sidra exactly how he feels about this memory as he's told this story. But he doesn't stop there. He finishes speaking by saying, "Just getting to watch you do both of those, side by side, was a real joy for me." In doing so, he has put the emotions that flowed through his body and out of his eyes into one simple word.

Does Ben need to explicitly name his emotion as joy? Hasn't Sidra already witnessed his joy being expressed in various other ways? There are many nonverbal ways for us to convey our emotions and all of them can serve as valuable, powerful points of connection when communicating with our partners. Words are just one method for articulating our love. While I would never want to suggest they're the most important or the most effective, just watch the way Sidra reacts when Ben says the word *joy* out loud. The loving expression with which she was already looking back at Ben—eyes welling up with happy tears and a closed-lip smile—splits open. In the instant that Ben articulates his emotion, her smile unfurls and spans her whole face. She even moves backward half an inch, as if she's been hit with the force of Ben's voiced joy and overtaken by it.

Although even in a conversation—an interaction that's built principally out of words—there are a lot of different ways to share our feelings with our partners, why not strive to hone the skill of emotional articulation so you can give your partner the same gift Ben was able to give Sidra? Getting the hang of emotional articulation may feel uncomfortable at first, but think of acquiring this skill as an act of service you're doing for your partner and for everyone in your life. Putting words to our feelings can be one of the greatest gifts we can give each other. But if you ever find that there are simply no words that you can find to hold your feelings, a simple moment of connected silence is articulation enough. Hold your partner's gaze. And let your emotions flow across the space between you.

II: The 12

These are the 12 questions that I've seen consistently deepen the connection between intimate partners; and, crucially, why and how they work. My intention is for you to read through this book, then refer back to these questions before starting an intimate conversation of your own with a partner by alternately asking one another each question. If you get stuck at any point, see Troubleshooting (page 174).

What are your three favorite memories we share and why do you cherish them?

You and your partner are about to step into a cathartic conversation, one that at times might feel like riding out a storm of emotions, being awash in the pure joy of your connection, doing open-heart surgery on your relationship, or all of the above, all at once. Yes, it can be a lot. So, before diving into the depths of your connection, it's important to remind yourselves why this relationship exists in the first place. While certain qualities may attract you to a partner, it's the experiences you created together that form the foundation of any relationship. By reliving those experiences together, the love and trust upon which your relationship was built are brought front and center, fortifying your connection for the new experiences that are yet to come.

A tree is only as strong as its roots. The deeper down into the earth those roots go, the taller the tree can grow and the more resilient it becomes to the elements. A conversation between partners is no different. If it's been firmly grounded in the love and trust out of which a relationship has blossomed, it will have a strong enough foundation to sprout expansive branches, stretching into uncharted, unexplored, and even uncomfortable territory while still maintaining the ability to weather any storm that might arise.

This first question serves to anchor the relationship in a positive space by reinforcing the connection between you and your partner, reminding you both how deep and intertwined the roots of your relationship have grown by virtue of the cherished memories you've created together.

Traveling Back to the First Sparks

The conversation you are about to have has been carefully designed to trace the journey of your relationship from where it began, all the way into a future you dream of having together. This question asks you to venture back into your shared past, retracing the memorable steps you have taken and created that have led to today.

A relationship exists in a continuous push and pull between the past and future. It starts at point A, with partners falling in love, and, for as long as it lasts, moves toward a distant point Z—the hopes and desires for the future that those partners share—with many points in between. But Point Z will never actually be reached, at least not until the relationship ends. As a relationship and each person in it changes on their own journey through life, new dreams and plans will continue to arise, pushing that point Z ever further into the future. Therefore, your relationship is always floating somewhere in between those two points—where you started and where you're heading. And this middle space is in constant flux as well. It's like a vast sea, filled with waves of experiences, challenges, and adventures upon which the relationship sails. You move over it, but it itself is in motion, speeding you up, slowing you down, and altering your course on your shared journey.

Although point Z will always lie beyond the horizon and where you are right now changes from moment to moment, the relationship's point A is stable, rooted in the fond memories you created and share. Think of it as the beautiful seaside town from which you set sail together. As you sail through the present, buffeted by change and life's rogue waves, thinking back to that town can be more than just a comfort; it can be both a grounding and a guiding force for you and your partner as you continue on your adventure.

To better understand where you are and where you're going, it's important to remember where you've come from. And that's not necessarily easy to do in your daily life. Surely the sea you've been sailing together has carried you far from wherever you started. Your relationship is different than it was when you first fell in love. Maybe the sea has calmed; it's become more relaxed or, perhaps, steadier than it once was. Or, maybe you're currently sailing high seas, a raging ocean with huge waves, which is proving exciting or terrifying or both at once.

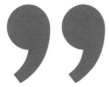

Something about you reminds me of being human . . . the most beautiful parts of being human.

—Gabrielle

"Dating After 8 Years of Friendship"
Scan here to watch the conversation

Regardless of where you are now, it's been a journey with a trail littered by the memories only the two of you, by virtue of your synergy, could create. Going back to the beginning and seeing how far you've traveled together builds trust between partners. Additionally, it is an acknowledgment of your connection. You've created moments that would not have been the same with anyone else. Your distinctive connection has created a synergy resulting in memories that are as unique as a thumbprint is to your relationship. With all the storms and doldrums of life, it can be easy to forget what specific possibilities exist because of your union and what solidified your love with the person you now share your days with. Because this question asks you to focus on your most cherished memories, it highlights to you and your partner what's only been possible because you have shared space and time together, and in effect solidified your connection to stand up tall to this present moment in time.

When you answer this question, you may find that the three memories you choose to share are different from those your partner selects, or that one of you is reminded of a wonderful memory they had forgotten until the discussion this question provoked uncovered it. Have fun together as you help each other fortify the foundation of your love by reliving these moments of connection. And keep in mind that the kind of memories you have created together speaks to the kind of memories you will and do create together. Your unique union creates a synergy that has that power to turn any moment you share into a cherished memory both of you will look back on fondly. Who knows? This very conversation could become one such memory.

When we have participants return to {THE AND} for a second or third conversation, we usually have them ask this question in each of their sessions. Almost every time, the memories they select are different. Although this question is about the past, allow it to also be a reminder that you and your partner are always creating memories. Reveling in these cherished moments is a reminder that new memories, every bit as sweet, are constantly being birthed.

Kat & Christina: Rewriting Laughter into Your Own History

A beautiful exploration around this question arose during Kat and Christina's conversation from {THE AND}. Married for five years, the two young women had a wealth of wonderful memories to choose from.

After Kat asks the question, Christina's brown eyes widen behind her glasses. Then she squeezes them tight, her long braids framing her face as she searches for moments she wants to share.

"It's hard because there's so many!" she says, tapping her long nails against her chin as she thinks. Kat laughs and leans her shaved head back, giving Christina the space to search their shared past. I bet that Kat is also running through a compendium of their shared experiences, curious about the ones her partner will choose.

"I think the memories I'm going to pick are the ones that made me laugh," Christina decides. She recounts the time they almost accidentally broke into a house together and immediately, upon telling the story, the laughter Christina experienced in that bygone moment is transferred to Kat in this present one. Kat cracks a huge smile and starts to giggle, reliving their misadventure.

"Finding out I was pregnant with Jackson," Christina continues. "That was surreal. Seriously, I was like, 'Hey!' It really does happen. Egg and sperm. I was like, 'Wow! Cool!'" Again, she has Kat laughing, and this time Christina joins in too. It looks to me like with each subsequent memory they share, their connection is growing stronger and stronger. They're beginning to mirror each other, laughing at the same time, tilting their heads to the same angle, sharing bright, brilliant grins.

"OK, that's two." Christina stops to think. "Maybe that long trip to New Jersey that took two or three hours to see that house and [we got] lost in the cornfield. And then taking some strange ride from a stranger and wondering if I was going to get killed." Once again, Christina's story elicits laughter from Kat. But this time it's laughter of disbelief. Kat's eyes have widened in shock. It seems to me like she's

QUESTION 1: What are your three favorite memories we share and why do you cherish them?

61

thinking that this wasn't a particularly positive or cherished memory, at least not for her. It was a scary one.

"Wow," she says, expressing her surprise that this is a memory Christina apparently adores.

"Because I was with you it was fun!" Christina explains. "And we survived." Kat takes a moment to look down. She nods. She smiles. Has an experience she had always remembered in a negative light just been completely reframed in such a way that it's now a source of laughter and joy for her? Did hearing her partner's perspective on her own history just allow her to rewrite it?

The Value of a Second Perspective

Our past is a collection of moments we recall. But how consciously aware are you that you are creating and building memories as those moments occur? Sometimes it takes someone else to reflect them back at you to remind you of the richness of the life you've lived. One of the greatest gifts of any relationship is that you move through life with a partner who helps record, and provides a different perspective on, the most important moments in your life.

Just look at what happened between Kat and Christina. Christina's perspective on their shared past had an effect on the emotional content of Kat's recollection of an event. We can't know for sure, but maybe now that she has a more complete understanding of how her partner experienced that event, Kat's memory of it has been forever changed. I've certainly seen this happen in my own life quite a lot. My brother— just fifteen months younger than me—has been one of the greatest gifts my parents gave me for this very reason. Because of our closeness in age, he's been present for so many important moments I've lived through. Whenever I hear him retell one of our shared experiences from his perspective, it always colors my memory of it with new emotional content and details that simply hadn't existed for me before. Suddenly my past has more depth, more context, and more meaning.

As incredible as it is to create new memories with the people we love, isn't it amazing that by reliving our old ones aloud with them, we end up recreating them as well? If we see our lives, our identities even, as an accumulation of experiences, then the richer and more vibrant our memories of those experiences are in our minds, the richer and more vibrant our lives can become. Furthermore, our memories change over time. And by talking them out with our partners, we are able to notice the places in which our respective recollections of the past have diverged, and thus, the things that are most important to each of us. What we choose to remember says a lot about what each of us most values.

Suggestions for How to Process This Question

Sometimes when this question is asked, participants struggle to find the right memories to highlight. They wrack their brains looking for the perfect experience—the fondest memory, or the most profound moment. But try to remember that there is no right answer to this question. Whatever memories that come up are the right ones for this conversation right now.

If you find yourself having a hard time deciding on a memory, try dropping into deep listening. Let go of trying to think about what story you want to share and bring your focus to your emotions. They will guide you to the resonant three memories most fitting for the exact moment this conversation is taking place.

QUESTION 1: What are your three favorite memories
we share and why do you cherish them?

63

What was your first impression of me and how has that changed over time?

Often, we fall in love with our first impression of our partner, with that initial story we tell ourselves about who they are. When this happens, it's not uncommon for the rest of the relationship to become a conversation with, and a challenge to, that original story that first drew us in. It's like an anchor we then pull against as the sea on which we journey through our lives inevitably carries us toward change.

That first impression that attracted us to our partner is lasting, for better or for worse. And yet, no matter how powerful a first impression remains, it lives only in your mind. Your partner has undoubtedly changed since your first meeting, and so have you for that matter. You aren't the same people who fell in love once upon a time. But are you holding on to the ghosts of those two lovers? Is that anchor to the past keeping one or both of you from growing into new versions of yourselves? What was your first story of who this other person was and how is that story changing for you as you each grow together and individually?

Flowing with Change Versus Swimming Upstream

As you live your lives together, the unfolding narrative of your relationship is constantly challenging the first impression of your partner. Revisiting it puts it in stark contrast with the person sitting in front of you, allowing you to see the path of change they've been walking from a holistic perspective. Perhaps certain aspects of how your partner changed were incremental as they occurred. Maybe you barely noticed them or took them for granted. Or perhaps you didn't want to acknowledge those changes because they are moving further away from the version of the person you were first attracted to. Some of us, or some part of some of us, wants to keep everything exactly as it was, and for it not to change at all. As you respond to this question, you have the opportunity to explore all the changes that your partner has undergone in their totality, making you cognizant of how each of

QUESTION 2: What was your first impression of me and
how has that changed over time?

65

you change as individuals. It allows for both of you to be able to live in the relationship's ever-changing present moment versus swimming upstream toward the past.

As you speak that initial image of your partner back into existence, you'll naturally begin to ask yourself questions about how you have been relating to that image—this person who is gone but might still occupy a lot of real estate in your mind and your heart. Is that the person who you're still in love with? Are you holding your partner up to the standard or story of the person they were rather than cherishing the changes that have made them into who they are now? Are they changing in a way that's destructive, one that might be ameliorated by your conscious awareness or intervention?

Or is the way they've changed over time the thing that makes you most proud of them? Perhaps noting these changes out loud will give you the opportunity to show your partner you've been aware of their bravery, their strength, and their growth for some time. Have you told them that lately? Could now be the perfect time to offer them that kind of empowering acknowledgment?

Whatever they might be, allow your expanding awareness of the changes you observe to build further trust between the two of you. They are proof of everything you've been through, signposts and landmarks on the journey you're on together, reminding you that what is the case today may not be the case tomorrow and vice versa.

Cat & Keith: Seeing the Difference

When Keith asks Cat how he's changed during their conversation for {THE AND}, Cat lifts her eyebrows, taking in the present version of her partner sitting across from her. "A lot," she responds, regarding her partner's close-cropped hair, ears pierced multiple times, and attentive green eyes that match his green button-up and tie. "A lot."

"

I feel like our relationship is the bedrock of my life."

—Ben

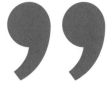

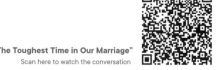

"The Toughest Time in Our Marriage"
Scan here to watch the conversation

A subtle flash of pride flutters across Keith's face as he takes in Cat's acknowledgment of his long and complicated journey. Cat leans into that, elaborating, "You know, physically, because of [you] transitioning from female to male." Her voice trails off here. Clearly she is about to elaborate further and sensing that, Keith leans in toward her, curious about what changes she's noticed that maybe he hasn't seen in a mirror. "You've always had passion for your work," Cat continues, shaking her head of black hair back and forth as she waits for the words to come to her. "But I think it's even more now. I think you're really, really, a real businessman now . . . And, look, you love that."

A huge smile spreads across Keith's face as Cat shares how she perceives him. How must it feel for him to have his partner say aloud that she's watched him grow into a version of himself that he loves? From his expressions, it seems like he's experiencing a real sense of relief from hearing that his transition hasn't just been a physical one, that now the true Keith is able to be seen and noticed by the outside world in a way that it hadn't before.

"I'm glad to hear you say that," Keith says. "Sometimes I don't know if you see the difference."

Keith and Cat show us how noticing and discussing the way someone has changed can be an empowering gift. If we're working on ourselves, endeavoring to show the world a kinder or stronger or truer version of who we are, it's not always easy to know whether we're achieving our goals. The eye cannot see itself. But when our partner, often our closest confidant, honestly tells us that yes, we are growing, we are changing, we are becoming the person we want to be, isn't that a relief? Isn't that the best encouragement there is to keep moving forward?

But this question can create the opportunity for far more than an acknowledgment, and Keith and Cat's powerful interaction shows us that as well. As they continue to discuss Keith's transition and the changes he's undergone, the issue of what might happen if more of that change doesn't occur or doesn't happen fast enough arises. Cat offered Keith empowering encouragement to continue down the path he's on, but what would happen if he stopped moving down that path? What would happen if he were to choose a different one?

"I have expectations according to my past relationships," Cat tells Keith. "Just the way things played out. The way people transition. The way they do things. So I have fear, sometimes, that it's not going to happen. Or that I'm going to get impatient."

As she's said this, Keith looks at Cat intently, nervously moving his hands around, his eyes wide as saucers. He leans forward, fully attentive, nose flushed red in anticipation. It looks like Cat isn't the only one with fear around this topic. Is Keith thinking Cat is about to give him an ultimatum? Some sort of timeline his transition needs to follow if their relationship is going to have a future?

"But," Cat goes on, "even if it doesn't happen, I still want to be with you. And you should know that."

"I didn't know that," Keith says. The nerves and fear that looked like they'd been building up inside him give way to a deep sigh of relief and watery eyes. "Thank you for telling me that. I didn't know that."

You can already see that this moment of communication and clarification has opened the door to new possibilities in their relationship that didn't exist prior.

The Constant Discovering of the Other

Change is such a powerful force in life. In fact, it is the only constant. The only guarantee in life is that things change. And the only time change isn't happening is when we are dead. It can hold the reins of our expectations. It can fill us with nostalgia or gratitude or anger or relief. But noticing how it has entered your life and your relationship will also allow it to increase your understanding of your partner and of humanity as a whole.

QUESTION 2: What was your first impression of me and how has that changed over time?

69

The passage of time and the subsequent deepening of your knowledge of your partner's growth can often recontextualize the moments you've shared. Paying attention to and appreciating this process can give you yet another reason to be thankful for the way your impression of your partner has changed the more you've gotten to know them. Reflecting on events you thought you understood at the time can suddenly offer you a surprising or nuanced perspective on a shared memory.

Here's an example that may sound familiar to you. In the beginning of a relationship, your partner tells you an anecdote, something about them. A year later, they tell you that same thing again. When they retell this story, you might think, *Well, I've already heard that, you're just repeating yourself.* Yes, indeed you have, but the meaning of the anecdote has changed because your understanding of the person relating it has too. Suddenly you're able to see a clearer and fuller version of your partner acting out their story in your mind's eye because you have a greater understanding of the context and who they are. What meant one thing then means something else now. A simple example is if on your first date you went on a roller coaster and had a great time. Then, a year later you learn that your now-partner is entirely scared of roller coasters but put on a brave face to make a good impression. Now their action on that first date takes a whole new meaning. They faced their fear. What seemed like a simple good time was actually them bravely facing their fear in order to connect with you. Now you can appreciate that action a lot more than you initially did.

Human beings are rarely as simple as we appear. It takes time and the building of real intimacy to peel back the matrix of layers we all carry with us. Your first impression of someone is the thing that draws you in, but how you relate to that impression can change, deepen, and expand over time. Are you cognizant of that process? Are you riding the wave of change in perception of the person you are with? Are you constantly rediscovering them anew? In the most vibrant, romantic relationships, partners try to stay conscious of the ever-changing person they're with by being present to their constant discovering of the other.

Suggestions for How to Process This Question

As these questions and the emotions attached to them come up for you, observe them gently. Have you been fighting against your partner's natural inclination toward change by wanting them to stay the way they used to be? Or, on the other hand, does seeing the way your partner has grown into themselves fill you with joy? Allow this to be an opportunity of awareness of whether or not you're trying to hold on to the past or surfing the present.

Change is natural and inevitable, something to cherish, and a reminder of how far you've come together. Therefore, try to look at the changes you notice in a curious and objective way versus making value judgments. You might be surprised at what you find if you sit in gentle awareness of these changes rather than rush to judge them. As your partner has aged, you might feel insecure about being attracted to your partner's body in a way you once were. But perhaps the unique way that they have grown into themself holds even more attractiveness for you, a beauty that is specifically precious to your eye as you behold it. Maybe your partner used to earn a lot of money and now that they have decided to pursue a less-lucrative yet more emotionally fulfilling dream of theirs, certain things in your relationship have become more difficult. Notice if their decision to follow their passion makes you proud or if it causes you to hold resentment toward them, and then sit with whichever emotion that observation generates within you. Try to remember that each change you notice is simply a reality of who your partner is now. There is no going back. Can you accept that? Even better, can you cherish it?

QUESTION 2: What was your first impression of me and how has that changed over time?

71

When do you feel closest to me and why?

Over the course of this conversation, you and your partner will revisit, reimagine, and discuss some of the pivotal moments in your relationship. At the beginning of the conversation, you'll each have shared three specific memories that are cornerstones of the love you've built together. You both picked those memories because they stick out in your mind as special. But, by nature of their specialness, they are aberrations—things that don't happen every day or every week.

As important as it is to cherish the big stuff—those pillars of your love that keep it standing tall—the mortar that holds a relationship together through life's ups and downs is made of much smaller moments. These recurring doses of intimacy are what keep you bonded. Sometimes they can be so small that you don't even realize they're happening as they occur. Just like some of the simple yet sweet moments in life, they can pass us by before we've even become aware of them. And this is where mindfulness comes in. As cliché as it may sound, stopping and taking the time to notice the sensation of the sun on your face, the taste of a sip of water when you're desperately thirsty, or the magical beauty in the dance of a campfire's flame can be the difference between deeply embracing life's richness and letting it slip through your fingers. A relationship is no different. Whether it's a weekly tradition of movie nights, a kiss that comes at the end of a long day, that one absurd inside joke that always leaves you both in stitches, or even just washing the dishes together after a home-cooked meal, these simple moments can be the most powerful points of connection between partners. It's those moments of shared conspiracy that are the mortar in the wall of your connection.

This question is an opportunity for you to zero in and identify those simple moments of closeness, to mindfully bring your awareness to a level of intimacy so deeply integrated into your relationship that it's easy to gloss over in spite of its connective power.

Finding Your Unique Connection Hiding in Plain Sight

The first two questions in this conversation have slowly brought you and your partner out of the past and into the present moment of your relationship. As we approach the here and now that you inhabit together, this question brings you out of a reflective mode and into one of mindful observation. Notice that the question is asking *When do you feel closest to me?* rather than *When did* or *When have you felt closest to me?* The idea here is to look for moments that recur, that unfold again and again in your daily life. This is an opportunity for both of you to see the relationship in action and to explore how that action keeps you bonded day in and day out, no matter what waves the sea of the ever-changing present throws your way.

Just as each relationship, each life, and each person are unique, these moments are yours and only yours. No matter how repetitive or banal they may seem on the surface, woven into their simplicity is the singular beauty of the intimacy you share with your partner. Even if your answer is something rather obvious, like, "When we make love," pay attention to why you chose that moment and you'll see that it's the specific details braided into the recurring moment you selected that trigger your feeling of closeness to your partner. Those details are unique to your connection. They wouldn't be there if you'd shared that moment with anyone other than the person with whom you're having this conversation. As you answer this question, let the sharing of those moments tug at the threads of your specific expressions of intimacy, pulling them out of the tapestry of your relationship for closer inspection. The intricacies in a human connection are easy to miss when you aren't looking closely, but they are what give it its strength and vibrancy. Revisiting these little moments together will remind you and your partner of what's special between you and of just how simple it can be to strengthen that bond with a new stitch at a moment's notice.

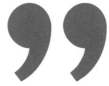

"

You
are
home
to me.

—Rafa

"Polyamorous and Monogamous Love"
Scan here to watch the conversation

Regardless of the changes you and your partner noted in each other as you answered Question 2 (*What was your first impression of me and how has that changed over time?*), these moments of intimacy you are now discussing continue to occur in the life you share. Thus, let this question be a way of demonstrating that despite whatever changes you each have undergone, the possibility to have regular instances of intimacy not only still exists, but it also continues to be activated by your relationship. The unique lines that make up the thumbprint of your love are still there.

Maddi & Martin: Making the Moment Theirs

Maddi and Martin had been dating for a little over a year when they sat down to have a conversation filmed for {THE AND}. They're both young and share a similarly open, inviting smile, and nearly identical shades of light brown hair—his, long and curly, hers, short and wavy— and pale blue eyes. When Martin asks Maddi this question, she takes a long, deep breath. You can see her rifling through her mental catalog of moments with Martin, searching for the one she wants to share. It doesn't take her long to find it, and when she does, she starts to giggle. "It's kind of weirdly specific," she says, through her laughter. "And usually you're asleep."

She goes on to tell Martin that after they've had a fight or a difficult experience together and have fallen asleep on opposite sides of the bed, not feeling particularly connected, she tends to wake up in the middle of the night. In that moment, she realizes that the fact Martin is still there beside her is far more important to her than whatever their conflict had been about. That's when she feels closest to him, in a private yet powerful moment of reconciliation, watching as her partner sleeps on.

"I'm like, what were you thinking?" Maddi says, recounting the way she'll speak to herself in the moments of realizing that their conflict is nothing compared to their love. Martin's attentive look splits open into a smile. "Why would I waste time [turning my back to you] when we could have been cuddling?" Maddi continues, mirroring her partner's grin. She explains that having felt the strength of their connection transcend whatever rift had come between them, Maddi will then carefully snuggle up to Martin, trying not to wake him.

Judging from Martin's reaction, it looks to me like she isn't always successful and that Martin remembers being woken up at night for a conciliatory cuddle on more than one occasion.

"Yeah," he responds, "I like it when it's like the middle of the night and then you just kind of"—he stops speaking and mimes out his interpretation of midnight spooning. From the excitement in his eyes, I feel like while he might have appreciated those moments as they'd happened, now, after listening to Maddi's response, his understanding of the depth and importance of those moments has grown.

The two of them dive deep into this shared moment of closeness, describing it in detail—from the tiny bed that makes not cuddling almost impossible to the specific way in which Maddi reaches out for Martin, closing the distance between them. By articulating and giving voice to it, they've put it in a place where it can be acknowledged and appreciated. They've made the moment theirs, sharing and reveling in the unique intimacy of their connection.

Meditating on Your Intimacy

As we saw with Maddi and Martin's experience in the {THE AND}, the beauty of the moments that come up in response to this question is in their simplicity. They can be things that are so mundane that you hardly notice them. But start paying attention and you'll find them scattered throughout the life you and your partner share. One of my favorite things about this question is that once it's been asked, you'll start paying more and more attention to the moments in which this simple brand of intimacy appears. I'd be willing to bet that in the wake of this conversation you'll start to notice many more of them than you'd been able to think of when formulating your answer. What better way to strengthen your connection to your partner than by becoming more aware of the ways in which it's already alive and thriving in your daily life?

This process of developing a conscious awareness of the moments in which your connection to your partner manifests has a lot in common with one of the core gifts offered by mindfulness meditation. The feeling of peace that washes over you when you're meditating and all your thoughts finally stop may be a familiar one. Possibly you've felt it many times before in your life. But you never noticed it for what it was until you began to meditate and consciously bring your attention to the beauty of that simple sensation. In my experience, the more I train myself to notice that feeling while meditating, the more I start to become aware of the times I stumble into that same kind of peace in my daily life. Learning to notice and appreciate simple moments of intimacy will offer the same benefits: a stronger awareness of your connection to your partner and the ability to fortify that connection by creating new moments for you to share.

Suggestions for How to Process This Question

Maddi's reaction when Martin asked her this question is typical of how I've seen many participants respond to it in {THE AND}. Before speaking, they usually start by taking a deep breath as they begin to search for moments of closeness. With that inhalation, they are consciously or unconsciously dropping into their emotions and allowing their feelings to guide them to the moment they eventually share. There is a vulnerability here, and you can see it play out on the face of the one answering. It's amazing how quickly our emotions will show up for us when we call for them. And this question draws out an emotion that is endearing and sweet. Enjoy it.

I would suggest that when responding to this question, you commit wholeheartedly to deep listening, letting your head remain quiet and directing your attention to the emotions that arise from your heart as you explore your memories. Remember, just like in Maddi's experience, it's possible that a moment in which you feel closest to your partner is something that at face value seems trivial, or silly, or totally unexpected to you. If you think too much about which moment you would like to choose, there's a chance that you'll end up picking a moment that meets our cultural expectations around what actions are supposed to denote closeness instead of choosing the moment in which you, personally, specifically, feel closest to your partner. Remember, there are many ways to feel close. And fortunately, there isn't a way to do it right. There can be big moments and small moments, actions or words, but none of them change the sense of closeness that you feel. So let your emotions help you select the moment that feels right to you now, and you'll be sure to illuminate a special thread of your connection in this conversation.

Whenever I've seen participants struggle with this question, either they're trying too hard to find the right moment out of many that come up—which means that after having listened to their heart and found something to share, their head butted in and they started overthinking their decision—or they suddenly realize that they don't have very many moments to choose from. Maybe they realize they don't have any moments they can think of at all. If this happens to you, relax. There are two positive ways to look at this. First, if you aren't experiencing regular moments of closeness in your relationship, that's a clear sign that something is going on that could use addressing, sooner rather than later. Is the lack of small moments of intimacy in your relationship the symptom of a bigger issue you hadn't been able to see clearly until now? Isn't it better to have realized this than to remain ignorant of it? Could that realization be the first step toward having a relationship that better meets your needs? Noticing something's absence is the first step to bringing it into your life. And therein lies the second positive takeaway: if you've noticed that your relationship lacks moments of recurrent yet simple moments of intimacy, now you are aware enough to begin to actively create those moments. Is there a way to turn one of your shared interests into a weekly or daily tradition? Are there moments when you could gift your partner an unexpected touch or smile? Remember, these are the kinds of moments to bring up in response to this question: the simple things. There's no need to trip yourself up by looking for ambitious, explosive moments and realizing you can't think of anything that lives up to that standard. Practice focusing on the small stuff and being grateful for what you have.

If you keep your eyes open for opportunities to bring simple expressions of intimacy into your life, you're sure to find them. Whether you struggle to find moments to share, find yourself overwhelmed by how many there are to choose from, or just instantly and instinctively know when you feel closest to your partner, I encourage you to keep your eye out for and your heart open to as many of these little moments of closeness as you can find in your daily life. The more you find hiding in plain sight, the deeper your connection with your partner will become and the more it will be present for you both to behold in all its unique brilliance.

What are you hesitant to ask me and why?

Let's face it. There's always something you are hesitant to ask your partner. And that's probably exactly what you two should be talking about.

Remember Ben and Sidra, the couple we looked to as an example of emotional articulation at work? If you've watched their videos, it's probably clear to you that they have gotten very good at having intimate conversations and communicating honestly, fully, and effectively. I'd hazard a guess that a big part of how they achieved this is their willingness to face points of hesitancy or fear between them head-on. During one of their many conversations for {THE AND}, Sidra said this to Ben in pretty much the most direct and succinct way possible: "If I'm scared of something to tell you, that's kind of the signal that I need to tell you something."

• • •

While Question 1, 2, and 3 dealt with building the base of your loving relationship, reminding you of your trust and love for one another, Question 4, 5, and 6 really pull at the strings of how you both deal with conflict. If you're going to build a long-lasting, strong, profound romance, you're going to have to get good at leaning into conflict. Exploring points of tension, of hesitancy, allows you to uncover the areas of misalignment in your relationship. Avoiding them doesn't make them go away. In fact, the opposite happens. However small these seeds of conflict may appear, if left unattended they can sprout into larger, more cancerous growths that will eventually become impossible to ignore. If you don't hash out these issues now, at some point something will happen that will force you to face them, and when that occurs, they will be much more difficult to manage. The less you venture into these points of discomfort, the more they fester, taking up more space and becoming more difficult to untangle and extract without painful intervention.

A Caveat

Let me be clear. Fear of the discomfort caused by a difficult conversation and fear of physical or emotional violence perpetrated by an abusive partner are two very different things. If you feel fear come up for you around a point of conflict in your relationship, check in with yourself honestly. Ask yourself if these fears are centered on exploring a challenging topic of conversation or if they are fears for your psychological or physical safety.

Within the pages of this book, I am speaking specifically about the former type of fear—fear of broaching difficult subjects of conversation with one's partner in the interest of growing one's relationship. Learning to lean into uncomfortable discussions like these with your partner is like stretching. The more you do it, the easier it becomes. And if you stretch every day and lean into the pain a bit, your relationship will become more flexible and more resilient to stress.

Bringing It Out of the Dark

It's time to exercise your communicative muscles by leaning into a little discomfort. And I really do mean a *little* discomfort. This question doesn't need to explore a major conflict in your relationship. It's not necessarily something that's painful or the thing that keeps you up at night. Notice that the question is about something you are hesitant to ask, rather than something you are scared to ask. Not only is "hesitant" gentler than "scared," it also subverts the opportunity for a respondent to brush this question off by saying, "There's nothing I'm scared to ask you." Even in the strongest, healthiest relationships, there will always be a topic that someone is hesitant to broach. At this stage of the conversation, it's more important for you and your partner to warm up by exploring something that isn't particularly overwhelming, and in doing so prevent whatever particular issue you choose to share from growing into something that is.

What's also very interesting with this question is that as the other person is thinking about their response, inevitably you are thinking about yours. Meaning you are probably wondering, *What are they hesitant to tell me? It's probably* . . . And then, when you hear them say what they are hesitant to speak about, what if it isn't what you thought it would be? In that pause before they answer the question, the space is filled with possible spots of contention—the ones they are thinking about and the ones you think they are thinking about. It's interesting to discuss those as well, at some point sharing, "Funny you say that, because I thought you were going to say this." Thus, you have more threads to pull apart and discuss if you wish to. Not everything needs or even should be discussed all at once. I just want to elucidate for you that a number of threads may appear by virtue of each partner wondering what the other is hesitant to share.

In relationships, it's in the dark where things grow. Out in the open, in the light, is where you actively build your bond together. But in the places where that light doesn't reach, issues, frustrations, and dysfunction can sprout and spread all on their own. The less you look at them, discuss them, and shine the light of your attention on them, the larger they'll become. Hopefully, the previous three questions have reminded you of your love and unique connection. They illuminated the structure of your intimacy and trust. Consider the forthcoming discussion about something you're each hesitant to ask as an invitation for the two of you to carry that light into the unexamined darkness of your life and see what's been growing there while you might not have been looking.

I've seen many relationships in which partners prefer to leave things unsaid in an effort to maintain the status quo. While this can work for a time and be a survivable situation for many, it denies both partners the ability to fully express their whole self. It's an understandable desire to want to only show the most palatable parts of us to our partner, but filtering ourselves like this comes at a price. Just because you've hidden something doesn't make it any less a part of you. By not expressing it and exploring it with your partner, you are restricting the amount of yourself that your partner gets to experience. On the other hand, bringing those pieces of yourself out into the light, conscientiously naming them, speaking about them, and sharing them with your partner invites the whole of you into the relationship. This is a way of being that allows for a more fully alive, more fully emotional existence. It's akin to watching a film in black and white versus full color in 4K resolution.

So that leads us to several questions: Why, then, is there so much fear around sharing our whole selves with another? Why the preference to not shake up the emotional status quo? Why do we have this tendency to try to protect ourselves from actually feeling completely?

Is it because we're afraid those feelings might overwhelm us? Is it because they might be too painful? And if so, then is the amount of discomfort that you can handle commensurate to the amount of richness you let into your life?

• • •

What I've found in my own experience is that this discomfort and pain that we're afraid of is actually a façade. It's not that it doesn't exist, but that it's never as bad as you think. Whenever I'm feeling overwhelmed, waking up at night with anxiety about the things I have to complete and the responsibilities that require my attention, as soon as I just start doing, start taking action, my sense of anxiety fades. It always reaches a crescendo just before I spring into action and start confronting its source. But once I take it on and address it, the anxiety becomes manageable and nowhere near as overwhelming as I'd first thought and felt it was.

As you step into this next phase of the conversation, in which you'll begin by discussing this point of hesitancy and then let the following questions guide you into more pressing conflicts in your relationship, I'd like you to keep in mind that even one small step toward working on a source of discomfort is a way of alleviating the torment we experience around it. Leaning into these topics, gently and mindfully, will mitigate the sting of the experienced pain around any given issue bit by bit, while at the same time building trust between you and your partner.

Ivo & Kevin: A Pressure Release Valve and Reassurance

After twenty-two years of marriage, Ivo and Kevin have had plenty of practice nurturing and building their connection, growing more and more in sync over the years. They both wore pale-blue collared shirts and blue jeans in their conversation for {THE AND}, both sported big, well-tended beards—Ivo's dark and pointed, Kevin's bright red. But even after two decades together, when Ivo asks his husband this

"

If you're going to love, love. Have no fear.

—Jon

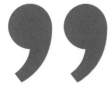

"Why We Seek Relationships"
Scan here to watch the conversation

question, Kevin immediately feels his way to the issue he is hesitant to bring up.

"Anything that's a trigger for you, for your anxiety and OCD," he shares, looking straight into Ivo's eyes. "Like, anything that has to do with problems with the house." Kevin then breaks eye contact as he goes deeper into how he has experienced the complexity of this issue alone, how he's kept it in the dark from Ivo. "I totally will keep it from you. Unless you find out about it first or when I do. Then I can't control it. But I will not let you know about a problem until I have taken it in, got my head around it, and have a resolution planned. Then I bring you in."

As Kevin shares this, it looks like Ivo is feeling conflicting emotions. On the one hand, he is seeing how his husband goes out of his way to protect him, but on the other, he feels the discomfort that this causes Kevin by overtly acknowledging their power differential out loud. Quickly, Ivo does the brave thing. He leans deeper into the uncomfortable moment, asking, "Does that make you resent me? Is that another burden in this relationship?"

"I've been resentful, I have"—Kevin begins before stopping short. His voice breaks. "Oh. Here come the emotions," he says bashfully as his eyes well up. Ivo smiles, and nods, his gaze radiating support and encouragement. "But because you're working on it," Kevin continues, "I know—I hope it's not always going to be that way."

Ivo smiles and nods as Kevin's acknowledgment of his hard work sinks in. Then, Kevin adds, his voice breaking once again, "But, it's—it's been a lot on me."

Ivo's eyebrows shoot upward. "To where you'd want to leave me?" he asks.

"No," Kevin says, authority and certainty back in his deep voice. He looks at Ivo and the serious expression that had come over his face melts into a smile. "Obviously not."

Here, this question has both allowed a point of discomfort in the relationship—the uncomfortable truth in which Kevin feels at times burdened by Ivo's disability—to be aired out, bringing it out of a place where it can fester into resentment and into the light. It has also given Ivo an opportunity to truly see his partner; he sees not only how Kevin has gone out of his way to accommodate him, but, more importantly, that Kevin is aware of his active efforts toward growth, and that ultimately that uncomfortable power dynamic is only one small aspect in the tapestry of their relationship. And then, right after Ivo watches the weight of this issue make his husband cry, he receives a verbal, unequivocal reassurance that Kevin's love for him is far more powerful than the issue itself. What a gift. From Kevin and Ivo's beautiful and courageous interaction, we see how this question can be both the opening of a pressure-release valve and a way of deepening understanding between partners.

The Right Time Is Right Now

When we realize that we are hesitant to talk to our partner about something, our natural tendency is obvious: we hesitate. Usually that hesitation is coming from a place of fear—fear of damaging the relationship or of hurting the other person or of seeming weak or needy or aggressive. And what happens next? Often, our minds then trick us into thinking that our hesitation is for a good reason. You might think to yourself, *You know, I need some time to think this through on my own before I bring it up with my partner."*

Whether that is an honest attempt to come to a difficult conversation more prepared or a trick of the mind to keep you from facing your fear, be wary of that impulse. Delaying an important conversation until the "right time" appears gives this issue more time to fester, more time for pressure to build, potentially making the conversation even more painful than it would have been had you brought it up right away. And while the impulse to think things through on your own may sound logical when it comes to relationship issues, it is almost always better to think them through out loud, as a couple, as a team. This isn't to say that one should never step away from a moment of heated conflict in order to cool down enough to be able to approach a future conversation with tact, calm, and an eye for the bigger picture. Waiting for those fight-or-flight feelings to pass is a productive, mature approach. However, if you take an honest look at yourself in a situation and find that you are taking the space because you are scared of discussing the confrontation or conversation, then yes, now is better than ever.

Consider how if you spend too much time thinking something through before you bring it to your partner, the conversation could start from a point of imbalance. Maybe you'll have already thought out everything you want to say and your partner has never even realized this is a point of conflict. They might feel blindsided if you recite your well composed yet rigid script at them. Maybe they'll feel like you haven't considered their need for how to process the information. Bring deep listening into the conversation and let the discussion flow from a place of trust and mutual understanding. Of course, there is a balance to be struck here. It's a good idea to give yourself some time to process an issue however it works for each of you. But while trying to get clarity in moments of quiet solitude can be helpful, true clarity will evolve out of the organic interplay between you and your partner.

So don't wait too long for the right time, because there's a good chance there never will be a right time. If you keep the tools from Deep Listening (page 42) and Creating a Safe Space (page 36) in mind, the right time is most likely right now.

• • •

When this question comes up for Andrew and Jerrold, a gay married couple of seven years, Jerrold—clean-cut, his short, dark hair connecting seamlessly with a short, dark beard—shares that he used to hesitate to share things that he felt might disappoint his husband. He admits that this came from a fear of losing Andrew, whose dazzling blue eyes soften at this statement. Jerrold goes on, explaining that his hesitance was motivated by a desire to protect a relationship he valued so strongly. But his hesitancy ended up having the opposite effect.

"It led to some pretty tough times with you not trusting me because I wasn't being completely forthright," he recalls. But by examining their relationship and how his behavior was affecting it, Jerrold realized that hesitancy wasn't the healthiest thing in his relationship. "I saw how it was hurting you. It wasn't beneficial. I wasn't being 100 percent with you. I have to give you my all in order for you to give me your all. And I don't want to hurt you. So, I changed. And now it's fine. Now I call it like it is."

Suggestions for How to Process This Question

Over the course of my life, I've learned that leaning into emotions like apprehension, tension, and nervousness can lead directly to an expansion of both skills and understanding. A few days before I launched my experience design studio, The Skin Deep, I got a call from my primary investor. He told me that he was going to have to pull his entire investment from the project. In the span of one extremely depressing phone call, I saw half of our total funding vanish. As I scrambled to continue pursuing my dream in the wake of what at the time seemed like a total disaster, I was repeatedly faced with situations that scared me on a visceral level. I'll never forget that feeling. On our first day of work, I remember taking a selfie with Heran and Paige, my first two team members, as we embarked on our adventure. Although I was smiling in the photo, inside, I was a wreck. But even as I was taking the picture, I knew I would always cherish that image, that I would look back on it knowing that in spite of how scared I was, I decided to move forward anyway with a smile on my face. And that's what I did. I kept moving forward, leaning into my fears anytime they came up. I quickly realized that I was learning so much, far more with things that seemed overwhelming or entirely unknown terrain. Soon, my ears began to perk up whenever I felt fear around having to do something I'd never done before. I'd go for it, seeing it as an opportunity for growth. If you look at the moments before your greatest achievements and successes, they were preceded by a strong dose of fear and apprehension. The act of persistence and courage are what transform a sense of fear into one of accomplishment.

Sometimes asking this question can be as scary as responding to it. But whichever end of it you're on, I'd invite you to sit in the pause that almost inevitably follows the asking of this question. In that moment, it can feel like anything can happen. Both you and your partner might be feeling nervous. But remember what came out of Kevin and Ivo's conversation around this question. Even though the issue they discussed was one that had caused Kevin a lot of discomfort, even though he expressed that discomfort emotionally and verbally to Ivo, together they reached a deeper, more complete understanding of the power of their love and the strength they each possess individually and share collectively. So breathe through that pause, sit in it for as long as you need, and then walk down that path of growth—which, remember, is lit by your fears—together.

What is the biggest challenge in our relationship right now and what do you think it is teaching us?

Every relationship has its challenges. No doubt about it. They're unavoidable, uncomfortable, and, I'd dare to suggest, invaluable. We don't grow in comfort; we grow in discomfort.

If you think you and your partner don't face any challenges, it's either because the small issues haven't grown large enough to be considered "challenges" yet, or because you're simply refusing to engage with conflicts that are there below the surface, sweeping them under the rug in order to stay in your comfort zone. Sometimes we spend more energy hiding away from facing the conflict than we'd need to spend actually dealing with it. The safe space you built as a container to hold this conversation was created so you can explore what lies beyond that cozy status quo, thereby expanding your understanding, skillset, and the expression of your full and embodied self. The courage to face the kinds of challenges that are outside the bounds of one's comfort zone and to then manage said challenges in a constructive manner is the key to any healthy relationship. Even more than that, doing so strengthens the roots that enable a sustainable, growing, and rich connection.

It's not the avoidance of conflict that teaches us how to be better and that makes us resilient; it's the ability to handle it constructively that speaks volumes to the flexibility and dynamism of a relationship. Therefore, the goal isn't to be free of challenges; it's to confront them with an open mind, to cherish them, make the most of them, and, once they've been resolved, welcome in the next one and all the teachings it can bring.

With this question, identify what each of you believe to be the greatest challenge you currently face. And, more importantly, to notice and embrace what it is you are learning from this challenge, from your partner, and from your relationship as it bends and flexes under stress. If you're not learning anything, you're missing out on what might be the greatest gift of sharing your life with someone else. Bringing the lessons inherent in a present struggle to the foreground of your awareness will show you what wisdom this challenge is trying to offer you.

Finding the Strength in Your Struggles

The previous question uncovered the seeds of challenges in your relationship by inviting you to lean into the discomfort that surrounds a point of hesitancy. Now that both of you have stretched those exploratory muscles, you're ready to do some heavier lifting.

Why is this question phrased so that it asks you to discuss your biggest challenge rather than your biggest problem? A problem is something that is inherently negative. It's something that you want to fix and then move on from as quickly as you can. But every challenge, no matter how difficult, is an opportunity. A challenge is something you face, overcome, and come out the other side stronger for having had it in your life. Going to the gym is a challenge you set for yourself in order to get stronger. It's not easy and it's designed to stress your system. But the more difficult your workouts are and the more often you show up ready to face that physical stress, the more resilient you become. Framing this node of discomfort as a challenge will make it feel more actionable and more like an opportunity to strengthen your bond.

The power of questions then serves to reframe this point of struggle in your relationship as a gift by asking you to each elucidate what you think the challenge is teaching you. This second part of the question places you in a space of a student, acknowledging that you have something to learn from it. And notice that the question has been worded so that it asks for what you think the lesson is, thus eliminating the possibility of "right" answers and acknowledging that both participants' responses will be subjective opinions rather than statements of objective truth. By asking you to look for the lesson you think lies at the heart of the challenge, the question takes the possibility of resenting your partner, or the challenge itself, off the table, creating a flexible and welcoming space in which to explore and to find teachings in your struggles.

"

When you accept love, you are also accepting pain.

—Avery

"

"Could I Have Been a Better Friend?"
Scan here to watch the conversation

Gabrielle & Luna: A Rewarding Quest Outside the Comfort Zone

When they sat down to have their conversation for {THE AND}, Gabrielle and Luna—two young people I'd assume were in their twenties— weren't officially in a romantic relationship . . . yet. Close friends since high school, they'd each separately informed my team that they had unspoken romantic feelings for each other. Ten months later, when they returned for a second appearance on {THE AND}, they'd fully opened themselves to each other and were in a romantic relationship. The fluidity in the way they communicated and the happiness that radiated off of them both in their second conversation was infectious, and I was filled with joy watching them ask each other questions and laugh together as they explored this new level of connection. But over the course of their first conversation, one could feel the elephant in the room of their unspoken feelings looming large over both of them.

Given their history, I wasn't the least bit surprised by Luna's answer when, during that initial conversation, Gabrielle asks them about the greatest challenge the two of them were currently facing in their relationship.

"Communication," Luna says with almost no hesitation. Luna has short curly hair, hazel eyes, and a silver ring looped through her septum. Gabrielle, sporting intense red makeup on her lips and around her green eyes, takes in her friend and smiles in response. Was she thinking about all the things she desperately wanted to communicate to Luna, but hadn't? And, by the way, this is often the most common response we see to this question. It seems to be the most prevalent challenge that comes up for most participants.

"I want you to tell me when you're upset, even when it's stupid," Luna continues. Suddenly, Gabrielle's face takes on a more serious expression. "Any little thing, like, 'Oh, you just said something to me and it pissed me off.' Tell me and we can talk about it and keep going. You don't have to bottle everything up until it just comes out over something tiny."

QUESTION 5: What is the biggest challenge in our relationship right now and what do you think it is teaching us?

97

Gabrielle nods and smiles again. "That's valid," she concedes. Then she offers her own answer to the question. "I think for me the biggest challenge is not something that is a challenge for you and I, but more for myself. And that's feeling like I can reach you." Now it's Luna's turn to give their friend a knowing nod. "A lot of times I do [feel that way]. Like you're just smoke; I can see you and you're there but I can't grab you and feel you in my hands." Again, Luna nods. Are they experiencing the same feeling? A desire to feel Gabrielle in their hands?

"I don't know," Gabrielle continues. "Sometimes it's just hard for me to admit things to myself. So I couldn't possibly explain things to you that I don't even know myself."

"It's whatever you're comfortable with—" Luna starts to say, but here, Gabrielle, swallows bravely, and cuts in.

"Have you ever been afraid of bringing something up because you feel like it would just make everything collapse under your feet?"

"Yes," Luna says, laughing and lifting her eyebrows a little. It seems to me that they know what Gabrielle is referring to, and that here they're acknowledging that they know, intimately, the shape of the challenge Gabrielle is facing.

Gabrielle smiles and nods. "Yeah, that's kind of what I've been struggling with lately."

"Well," Luna says, looking away, maybe wary of revealing their feelings first. "Whatever it is, you don't have to deal with it alone. Whatever your mess is, I'll make it my mess and we'll clean it up together."

They both burst into giggles, making eye contact and sharing a tender moment of connection.

This is as close as they got to sharing their romantic feelings for one another during their first filmed conversation, but I like to think that this was the seed that eventually grew into a full confession of love. Here we can see how talking about challenges and points of conflict can lead us to become who we hope to be, to have the lives we want to have. Out of a conversation about a lack of communication, two long-term friends began to break down the walls between them. It's clear from their body language, the way they look away from each other and trip over their words at times, that this wasn't exactly a comfortable topic for either Luna or Gabrielle to broach. But look at the reward it eventually brought them: a connected and long-desired romance. Would they have ever received that gift had they not bravely waded through this moment of discomfort, however awkward it might have felt? What would you rather experience: a brief sojourn out of your comfort zone or a lifetime of wondering what might have been had you only started to speak your truth?

Taking In the Lesson

It's tempting to tell yourself that if the one big challenge you're facing weren't there, everything would be fine. If only you had more of X, if only your life was free of Y, if only you could tell your best friend how you felt about them, you'd be able to be your best self. But the truth is, if every current challenge you were facing was suddenly erased, it wouldn't be long before a new one came into your life, offering you the decision to either fight against it or learn from it. This is why this question asks you to share your greatest challenge "right now." Tomorrow, or next week, or next month there will be another.

In the scope of a relationship, you may start off sharing a strong sexual connection with your partner, but the two of you are constantly struggling to make ends meet. Fast forward a decade and now your financial challenges have been overcome. Money is no longer an issue. But that sexual connection that was once so strong has waned. Your challenges have switched places, giving you something new to work on together. There is no finish line to cross where on the other side everything is smooth sailing. You overcome a challenge, and sooner or later a new one will appear. And, believe it or not, this is more good news. Because every single challenge you face is a new opportunity for learning and growth. But be careful. That empowering change will only truly be taken into your being if you actively look for the lessons in those challenges.

Maybe you've not only accepted that life is full of challenges, but you've also become an expert at overcoming said challenges. Wonderful. Great work. But the next, and far more important, step is to pay attention to whether or not you're truly assimilating the lessons each challenge has offered you. Becoming better at learning from your challenges won't stop future challenges from coming your way—that's impossible—but it will stop you from getting stuck in a cycle of facing the same challenge repeatedly, ensuring that all the hard work you put in whenever you face and overcome one will directly contribute to your growth. If you expend energy again and again working through the same challenge that appears repeatedly in your life, you probably haven't really learned whatever it is life is trying to teach you.

• • •

When I was in my twenties and thirties, I ran up against the same challenge in my relationships over and over again. Without realizing it, I used to exclusively seek out partners who had this impenetrable emotional wall up and who would run away from real intimacy. I found myself stuck in a highly unpleasant pattern in which I was always chasing after my partners, reaching and straining in an effort to truly get close to them. And on top of that, my low self-esteem placed my own self-worth on the response I got from my partners. If they responded positively, I felt high and worthy. If not, I was depressed. I was dependent on them for my own sense of well-being. It was not only frustrating, but also exhausting. Yet whenever any of them would stop figuratively running from me and actually give me the chance to build the kind of deep emotional connection with them I was certain I'd wanted, then I would turn tail and flee their overtures of intimacy. This exact same series of events happened so many times that I began to feel like a hamster running on its little exercise wheel, wondering why the scenery around me never changed.

Knowing what you already know about my family history, maybe you can guess where this self-defeating tendency that defined Young Topaz's love life came from. A combination of low self-esteem and a subconscious fear of the intimacy I desired but had no idea how to invite into my life kept me running in painful, frustrating circles. The only way I felt comfortable in a relationship was if there was an imbalance—that same lack of intimacy I'd seen modeled between my mom and dad—causing me to feel like I was always pursuing a deeper connection with my partner than they were capable of giving me. Their emotional unavailability allowed me to stay in my comfort zone, even though I experienced that "comfort" zone as extremely painful.

And if I did find a partner who was present and loving, believe it or not, I would get a stomachache. The same stomachache that my parents have told me I would get as a kid every time I moved between my parents' homes. And thus, I would take that stomachache as a sign this relationship wasn't right, when really it was just me not processing and facing the pain. The body remembers. The body keeps score. This is why deep listening—listening to your body and letting it speak through you—is such a powerful tool. I used to think that listening to my body meant that these physical pains were a sign that I should run, and therefore, I would end that relationship with the caring, present partner. I now see that this was just fear, which frankly lived in my stomach, reappearing and my body trying to protect me from having to face that fear of intimacy—the thing which I craved. Ironic right?

Out of this unhealthy dynamic, the same challenges arose again and again in these imbalanced relationships. Over time, I got very good at overcoming many of those individual challenges

QUESTION 5: What is the biggest challenge in our relationship right now and what do you think it is teaching us?

101

with a given partner and, on a surface level, things would get better between us for a while. But before long, new challenges would arise out of the same core issues and the vicious cycle would repeat itself. Those challenges were all trying to teach me the same lesson—*Stop chasing, stop running, and face your own fear of intimacy!*—but because I was so focused on solving each individual issue and moving on as quickly as possible, I never paid attention to that greater lesson.

It took a long time, many moments of uncomfortable self-reflection, and a profound and vulnerable conversation with a trusted friend before I was finally able to see the lesson this vicious circle of challenges was trying so hard to teach me. But when I did, I put all my energy into truly learning it, owning it, and facing my fear of intimacy head-on. As you might imagine, inherent in that process were many moments of flailing around far away from the padded furniture of my comfort zone. But once I accepted that path, sat with my discomfort, and faced my fears, I actually did change. I broke the cycle and was able to enter into more fulfilling relationships than I ever had before.

Suggestions for How to Process This Question

The best way to enter into difficult topics like those that may arise from this question is armed with a healthy dose of gratitude. Try to see this as an opportunity for you and your partner to learn the tools necessary for overcoming the next challenges you'll inevitably face and taking in their lessons fully, rather than as a venue for placing blame on one another. Remember that the challenge itself isn't reflective of either of you as people; it's reflective of the dynamic between you. And much like the memories you cherish are a synergy to your connection, so too the challenges and how you work through them can be unique to your connection. Recognize that. Articulate it. Be grateful for it. There is no need to get defensive, to feel attacked, or to do any attacking. Neither of you is defective or "wrong." It's the connection between you that may be experiencing a bit of dysfunction. With understanding, patience, and gratitude, fixing it together might be easier than you'd have thought. Or maybe not. Maybe the dynamic between you is irreparable and you'll decide to each go your separate ways, moving toward healthier and more fulfilling connections that would better resonate with each of you as individuals.

But that is an extreme outcome from facing a challenge together. Challenges are healthy and natural opportunities. As you sit with this question, remember that a relationship without any challenges is a death. There is no room for growth, learning, or deepening intimacy. Stagnancy is the opposite of living. The point is not to find out how to not have any challenges in your relationship, but to ask yourself, "Is this a challenge I'm OK to have?" What do I mean by this? Let me explain.

When I first started off traveling around the world and making films, having enough money to fund my projects and to just generally survive was a constant challenge. Facing it and finding ways to overcome it wasn't easy. But it was a challenge I was all right with facing and learning from, much preferable to me than the challenge of "I'm so bored with my life and have no passion in it." We all have challenges. In my case I was living a passionate, exciting, adventurous life; however, my challenge was financial. On the flip side, I could have had a day job in an office, and thereby no financial challenge due to consistent income, but then instead my challenge would be trying to feel passionate about what I was doing daily. There is a give and take to everything. So the question is not avoiding challenges entirely but understanding that one choice denies another and welcoming your challenges with gratitude.

If you run that same sort of analysis on the challenges that arise out of this question and take an honest look at the dynamic between you and your partner, what do you see? Are the kinds of challenges you face ones you're all right with facing? And are you paying close attention to what they're trying to teach you, allowing you to break unhelpful patterns and grow together? Are you finding the lesson that life is trying to teach you by allowing discomfort, that powerful teacher, your way? And once you've found it are you really letting it sink into your awareness, your actions, your being?

What is a sacrifice you feel you've made that I haven't acknowledged and why do you think that is?

Sacrifice may feel like a big, loaded word, but it's part of the balance of any healthy relationship. The beauty of being in a relationship is that you're invited to grow beyond the person you are when you're alone. In order to step out of the person you've been and into who you become while in connection with another human being, some sort of change—in behavior, personality, or priorities—may be required of you. Through this transformation you gain and learn a lot. It is a wonderful way to grow. But inherent in compromise and accommodation is also loss, which can be painful and, at times, breed resentment.

Sometimes our tendency can be to hide that pain from our partner, especially when that pain is directly caused by the relationship itself. But hiding a wound only stops it from getting treated. With this question, space is created for both partners to acknowledge a sacrifice each has volunteered in order to make the relationship work, one that hasn't been discussed before. Often you'll find that by simply acknowledging that sacrifice, the wound is healed and any resentment you or your partner might be harboring gets nipped in the bud.

At the end of the day, the sacrifices we make for our relationship, however challenging or painful, are gifts we offer to the relationship. But how can either of you see a sacrifice for the offering it is if you don't bring it into the light of your collective awareness? Answering this question is the time to do so.

A Leap into Discomfort—with a Bungee Cord Attached

Maybe when you're asked this question, what comes up for you doesn't feel big enough to be called a sacrifice. Maybe you don't want to give yourself that much credit or put that much emphasis on something that's painful to you. But this question has been worded like this intentionally. Even if you, personally, wouldn't call whatever you've done a sacrifice because that seems too extreme, it's important for both you and your partner to feel the weight, power, and beauty of these concessions, compromises, and selfless acts. Whether you'd normally call it a sacrifice or not, giving something up for your partner can be painful, or at the very least, lead you to start viewing aspects of your relationship as imbalanced. No matter how logical the reasoning or how willingly you do it, it can feel like a sacrifice. Just sharing and noting those points of disequilibrium gives each of you a more complete perspective on how each of you affect the other.

The next part of the question, *that I haven't acknowledged,* serves to shed light on something that has lived in the relationship's shadows until now. There's a good chance that this will be one of the bigger and more uncomfortable sacrifices you've made. Maybe there are sacrifices that your partner has acknowledged, but the ones that are most painful are the ones that we talk about the least, if at all. Having spent the last two questions practicing leaning into conflict, you're ready for a challenge. Again, the more willing you are to rise to the challenge that this question offers, the more rewards you'll reap from the conversation. This is especially true here. Often, the lack of acknowledgment stings far worse than the sacrifice itself. The line between sacrifice and gift can be quite thin. All that is required to shift an act from the former to the latter is appreciation. The simple step of finally receiving that acknowledgment can be enough to defuse any ticking time bombs of resentment that have been planted by an unappreciated sacrifice.

But until that recognition is given, it's natural to feel a lot of prickly emotions toward your partner while you discuss an unacknowledged sacrifice. I've found that it's far healthier to vent those emotions, especially while you're in a safe space to do so, than to let them fester unsaid. Doing this can be scary. Not only are you not sure how your partner will react, but you don't want to hurt them. Rise to meet that fear and know that the structure of this question has you covered. It might be uncomfortable at first, but it won't leave you and your partner stuck in an irreconcilable space.

The real beauty of this question is in the third part: *and why do you think that is.* Engaging with all three parts of this question will necessitate an answer in which you will try to better understand your partner and their motivations for having not acknowledged your sacrifice. This invites the partner who's carried a source of pain and resentment to step into their partner's shoes after having expressed it. In sharing why they imagine their sacrifice hasn't been acknowledged, space is created to build empathy and understanding—perhaps an understanding that has never been reached before this very moment.

Maybe as you talk through why your partner hasn't acknowledged your sacrifice, you'll realize that the situation reminds them of some trauma related to their childhood or that by recognizing your sacrifice they would have opened themselves up to a level of pain and vulnerability they'd been afraid to face alone. Looking deeply at this source of discomfort can help you uncover levels of rich complexity in your partner that you haven't seen clearly until now. It's not the space to heal from that trauma, but rather to explore both points of view, which allows each partner to be seen and transforms what was once resentment into a deeper understanding.

This perspective shift gives your response, however raw, a safety line—a bungee cord that will snap the conversation back into a place of compassion no matter how deep you dive into the emotions surrounding the pain your unacknowledged sacrifice has caused. While it's essential that we talk about these sacrifices, losses, and issues, there is nothing to gain in emotionally punishing someone you care about. The final part of this question gives you the immediate opportunity to show your partner caring and understanding, the best salve for any friction your honest venting has created. Of course, this only works in the absence of a relationship in which there are abusive, sociopathic, or manipulative dynamics. Begin from a place of equal love and caring for your partner and practice this ebb and flow of emotions—the airing of a grievance, followed by a loving dose of understanding—creates something invaluable when it comes to strengthening and maintaining connection.

Kat & Christina: Taking Pride in a Fierce Love

So far I've framed this question as a possible point of conflict, where repressed emotions and unspoken resentments around a sacrifice you've been holding on to get aired out before a moment of empathy reestablishes your connection. That can definitely happen here, but it's far from the only possible outcome of talking about sacrifices with your partner. Let's look again to Kat and Christina, the queer married couple whose conversation we touched on in Question 1 (*What are you three favorite memories we share and why do you cherish them?*), as an example of how this question can work almost in reverse—where one partner acknowledges a sacrifice the other has made, maybe without even realizing it, and that results in laughter and a greater sense of closeness between two partners.

When this question comes up, at first, neither of them can agree on who sacrifices more in their relationship. Both Kat and Christina think their partner is the one who carries the greater burden, and when either of them points out the sacrifices they see their wife making, both respond with surprise.

When Kat attests that Christina makes more sacrifices, Christina's eyes widen. "Now I'm curious. What do you mean by that?" she asks.

"You sacrifice your sanity for my habits—my cleaning habits—and my lack of order and attention," Kat explains, eliciting a burst of laughter from Christina. "I don't know," Kat continues. "I just feel like I don't really sacrifice anything, so therefore you sacrifice more."

"Can I tell you? I disagree with you," Christina playfully retorts.

"Really?" Now it's Kat's turn to widen her eyes in disbelief. "Why?"

"Your family are not exactly jumping up and down [shouting] 'Woohoo!' about you being with a woman, OK?"

I can see Kat really letting this sink in, considering it. She tells her wife that she feels Christina's endured the same level of disconnection from her family. But Christina's having none of it. She brushes

QUESTION 6: What is a sacrifice you feel you've made that I haven't acknowledged and why do you think that is?

109

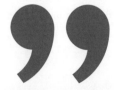

I love you because of how much you show me love . . . because you never stop even in the hardest of moments . . . the love that you give out, the love you show, is just always pouring even when I try to stop it, even I try to tell you I don't deserve it, it just always comes.

—Kadia

"I'm Scared of Going Bankrupt"
Scan here to watch the conversation

it off, saying "They already exclude me because I'm deaf." Then she returns the focus to Kat's family.

"In our relationship I saw how difficult it was with you and your mom," Christina says. Kat nods, conceding the point. "I'm sorry to bring this up again, but for the wedding your mom showed up late. She was supposed to walk you down the aisle. It says a lot. Your mom is still struggling [to come to terms with our relationship]. I feel like, daughter to mom, that relationship is so important."

Christina goes on to list several relationships in Kat's life that she's seen become strained or dissolve altogether as a result of Kat's decision to marry her. As she lists them out, Kat's face falls a bit. It looks like she's feeling the weight of those losses stacking up, seeing, maybe for the first time, that she's actually sacrificed a lot for her relationship. Then, Christina shares, "I just feel like how we deal with life is a little bit different. For me, I felt like maybe I was already at a disadvantage. Maybe I felt like, 'I'm black, I'm deaf, I'm a female, so what? I'm already down. So what?' But for you, it feels like I don't want to say you had to come down [to be with me]. You didn't. But you had a lot more obstacles being with me than I did with you."

Kat's smile here is priceless. It truly looks to me like she has never really considered the things she's had to give up for her relationship before. And when Christina acknowledges those sacrifices, I see pride in her willingness to put her love first flowing out of Kat's every pore. Maybe she's never realized just how important, just how sacred, her connection with Christina is to her. Maybe she needed to have her actions reflected back at her in order to really see the fierceness and strength of her love for her wife.

The Gift of Acknowledgment

If we look at what happened between Kat and Christina, it was Christina's acknowledgment of Kat's sacrifice that led to Kat being

QUESTION 6: What is a sacrifice you feel you've made that I haven't acknowledged and why do you think that is?

111

able to see the relationship from another perspective. The power of receiving a simple acknowledgment shouldn't be underestimated.

Remember Kevin and Ivo from Question 4 (*What are you hesitant to ask me and why?*), the gay married couple whose honest conversation around a point of hesitancy led to a tearful reaffirmation of their connection? Just after the point in their conversation where we left them, they begin to go deeper into exploring their conflict. After having gone back and forth over certain issues they didn't quite resolve, deciding instead to "agree to disagree," Kevin looks to me like he's carrying a lot of the tension of their conflict in his body. There's a moment of silence between the two in which he's smiling at Ivo, but I see it as a bit of a tight, forced, smile.

But just then, Ivo breaks the silence, telling Kevin, "You carry a bigger burden in this relationship than I do. I know that. And I appreciate it."

The changes in Kevin's physicality and expression as Ivo's acknowledgment hits him are monumental. All of that tension leaves him and a relaxed smile takes over his face. "Thank you!" he sighs, bowing forward as relief at the sacrifices he's made being recognized wash over him. "Thank you."

Feeling the acknowledgment your partner has yet to offer can be all you need to unwind tension that's twisted itself into the space between the two of you. In fact, just that simple recognition could be all it takes to transform your sacrifice from a point of pain to a point of pride. From the moment of acknowledgment all the way until the end of their conversation, I can see Kevin glowing with a sense of self-love and empowerment, having really been shown the positive effect he's had on Ivo through making uncomfortable sacrifices. Often, when you sacrifice something and it's acknowledged, you feel good because you're doing something for someone else. You're supporting someone else. You're giving a bit of yourself to a person you care for. Few things in life feel as inherently wonderful as that. But there's no better recipe for instant resentment than giving a gift that is unacknowledged, unappreciated, or downright ignored. It's the acknowledgment that can make all the difference.

What's also interesting is the relationship between this question and the two that precede it. Questions 4, 5, and 6 pull at the strings of how your dynamic contends with conflict. Question 4 (*What are you hesitant to ask me and why?*) is about hesitation, meaning it's about a seed that, if left unattended, will grow into what Question 5 (*What is the biggest challenge in our relationship right now and what do you think it is teaching us?*) explores: the biggest challenge. And Question 6 (*What is a sacrifice you feel you've made that I haven't acknowledged and why do you think that is?*) is about unacknowledged sacrifice, in which someone solved a challenge, but didn't receive the acknowledgment of the other. In other words, rather than try to tackle a challenge as a team, one person in the relationship found a way to solve it on their own, and thus bit their tongue and dealt with it, which can lead to resentment. So these questions are related in that they are dealing with the seed of possible conflict, the conflict itself as it is now, and a conflict that hasn't properly been resolved and has been left festering.

Suggestions for How to Process This Question

Take your time with this question. There are multiple layers to it and each one of them might be the catalyst for a cathartic and healing conversation between you and your partner. Go nice and slow. Don't feel like you have to rush on to the next question. Let everything that needs to come out, come out. Then let them respond. This can be a valuable moment in which you each learn something new about how your partner thinks through the interactions that cause friction between the both of you. Let this question work its magic, shifting the perspective on a point of conflict back and forth and back again. If you give it enough time, you might be surprised at just how much it can deepen your understanding of your relationship.

What is the pain in me you wish you could heal and why?

This is one of the most profound and challenging questions to converse around. We are all here having this human experience, a large part of which is the interplay of connection and disconnection, of integration and loneliness, of happiness and sadness. Pain and joy are the axis by which our experience of living and engaging in relationships, intimate or otherwise, pivots.

Part of life is incurring pain, and we tend to look to others, especially our intimate partners, to heal the pain within us. But in most cases, they can't heal us, and their well-intentioned but futile attempts to do so become the source of more suffering—suffering felt by both parties. While we are only really able to heal ourselves, that healing can be supported by those around us who hold the space for it to happen. Often, it is simply our partner's heartfelt desire to heal us that creates and nurtures that space.

In {THE AND} we often build to climax with this question, as this is the most vulnerable space we live in, and while exploring it can be challenging, it is often what solidifies the relationship. On the one hand, for the most part, you want to be healed by your partner. On the other, for the most part, your partner wants to heal you but cannot. This question reveals the vulnerability of both parties: one's desire to heal, and the other's desire to be healed. It reveals the opportunity to support and to nurture, which inextricably links the two and may be the unconscious bedrock of the relationship.

You Know Each Other's Pain Intimately

In {THE AND}, this question usually goes down like this: a participant picks up the card and reads it, usually to themselves before reading it out loud. Emotions might start to run high even before they speak it aloud to the other person. They are already going to their pain, feeling not just its weight, but both the beauty in their partner's desire to heal it and the tragedy of their inability to do so. They usually know exactly what their partner will say. And once the question is asked, the respondent identifies and starts to feel their partner's pain in an instant. Even though it's not theirs, they still live it. They have it in them by association.

When this question came up during Maddi and Martin's conversation, even before Maddi verbally asks it, she tears up. She is already feeling her own pain and the pain Martin experiences in not being able to heal it for her. When she does ask the question, he doesn't even need to respond. Does he get emotional because he feels her pain, his own frustration, or because he feels her sympathy for his impossible desire to heal her? A whole universe of connection, understanding, and love interwoven between them is revealed as they simply sit there and gaze at each other through their tears. The stars in that universe, beautiful and bright as they are, are crystallized through pain.

This is something that is intrinsic to every relationship of a certain length and depth of intimacy: you know the other person's pain. You can feel it in your gut even though it's not yours. What does that say about us humans? What does that say about empathy? And how does your sense of your partner's pain change over time? Does the pain dissipate as you both get used to it? And what can we actually do to heal each other?

This is the emotional climax of the conversation you and your partner have been moving through together. Questions 1, 2, and 3 have built trust between you, reinforcing and reminding you of your shared love and appreciation for each other. Questions 4, 5, and 6 have been preparing you for the vulnerability necessary for facing this question with an open heart. Take a deep breath and step into it; you're ready for this.

Lynnea & Eliza: Becoming a Guide on Your Partner's Healing Journey

Emotions had been running high from the very first question Lynnea and Eliza asked each other during their conversation for {THE AND}. A couple of nine years, from the way they interacted it looked to me like they'd been through a lot together. But when Eliza—wearing a backward black and red ball cap, black T-shirt, red shorts, and matching red basketball shoes—asks what pain Lynnea wishes she could heal in Eliza, the door is opened for an even greater depth of emotional truth to enter their conversation.

The instant Eliza finishes asking the question, Lynnea, whose rainbow-dyed hair and tie-dye dress contrast completely with her wife's athletic outfit, is ready to answer. She knows the heaviest burden Eliza carries without a doubt, and she responds immediately.

"The loss of your mom." She shakes her head, and it looks to me like she's feeling the weight of that loss pressing down on both their shoulders. "I really do [wish I could heal it]," Lynnea continues, "but I know I never can."

Throughout their conversation Eliza has bravely allowed her emotions to flow through her. She's laughed and cried freely with an open heart whenever she's felt moved to do so. But faced with a topic this painful, she lowers her sunglasses over her eyes. The muscles in her face strain to contain her hurt. It looks like it's simply too big for her to let herself feel completely.

"What I want you to do [is] heal it yourself," Lynnea goes on, biting her lip as she watches Eliza. "Because no one can heal your pain." The expression on Lynnea's face seems to say that she knows this isn't what either of them want to hear, but that it's the reality nonetheless. Maybe the idea of healing herself feels overwhelming to Eliza. How would she do it? Where would she even start? As she'll go on to say in just a minute, Lynnea wants to be able to take on the process for Eliza.

But she knows she can't. Healing this pain is Eliza's challenge, one only Eliza can overcome.

So what does Lynnea do? She tries to give Eliza several perspectives on processing that pain she feels might be useful on her partner's journey toward healing.

"I just want you to understand what happened while [your mom] was here," Lynnea says, beginning with a logical point of view. "You know, she was sick, babe. It wasn't like she was murdered or something like that. She died of a sickness that she fought for years."

Then Lynnea shows Eliza the cost of holding on to her pain. "And you put your college career on hold, put it all the way on the back burner and forgot about it . . . to take care of your mom." Lynnea's words catch in her throat as she says this and connects to the excruciating sacrifices Eliza has made. It's only now, when Lynnea's emotions start coming through, that Eliza lets go and begins to cry. Is she crying because she's seeing the way her suffering is reflected back to her through Lynnea? Is Eliza simply moved by the strength and solidarity of their connection? Or is she clearly seeing the way her pain haunts not just her, but her relationship, how it inhabits the space between her and Lynnea, causing all of these feelings to rise up inside of her all at once in a beautiful swell of catharsis?

"I don't think nobody comes back from losing a parent, especially a mom," Lynnea continues, "but if I could, I would take it. I would take your pain . . . Because you already know how I deal with hurt. I don't let it kill me. That ain't what you're supposed to do. You're supposed to take your lessons, whether it's good or bad, whether it's a loss or a gain, you just gotta take it and learn how to live with it because that's yours and it's never going to go away. I just want you to learn how to live with that wound without it [breaking] you."

Even faced with the fact that she can't make Eliza's pain disappear, what Lynnea has done here is take this opportunity to offer compassionate advice that she hopes will help her partner to learn to heal herself. What more can we do for our loved ones than this? To become an empathetic container for their healing, to let the relationship itself be the compassionate space in which they can find their own path to peace and do our best to hold the space for their journey.

Avoiding a Cycle of Suffering

As Lynnea points out, trying to heal our partner's pain is usually an exercise in futility. Even setting aside the near-impossibility of actually removing someone else's pain for them, would this really be the best thing for us to do? Or would it rob our partners of some of the most profound opportunities for growth and self-knowledge that life sets before us?

Furthermore, the act of trying, and probably failing, to heal our partner's pain for them usually comes at a cost. It becomes a source of more suffering, not just for ourself as we grapple with our own impotence, but for our partners as well. How would seeing that your pain is not only hurting you, but that it's hurting your partner as they struggle to fix something they have no control over, make you feel? Andrew and Jerrold touch on this in their conversation for {THE AND}. Andrew shares that in the past, witnessing Jerrold's well-intentioned efforts to help him get through his most painful moments would only make Andrew feel worse.

"One of the hardest things is having to tell you that there's nothing that you can do to help and then seeing how powerless that makes you feel and how sad it makes you look," Andrew shares. "It's just terrible because if I could make you happier I would. But there's just sometimes in life when nobody can help you and you just have to work through it." Luckily, they were able to break this cycle of suffering when Jerrold realized he "had to take all of the control out of it," step back, and let Andrew find his own way to healing.

But this doesn't mean that our partners can't help us at all as we try to move through our pain. In fact, they can be our most valuable resource of support as we learn how to heal. Maybe your partner sees the pain you refuse to see but feel regardless. Maybe your partner is seeing what you cannot see or something you can't quite look at because it's too painful. Whether you can see it or not, you experience it, that's for sure. The pain is so strong that you feel incapable of looking at it, because then you'd actually have to deal with it.

Think about the human body. What happens when you get physically injured? Your body pumps you up with tons of endorphins and adrenaline so that you don't feel pain. You are in shock. You can see your bone sticking out of your skin, but you don't necessarily feel it. That is your body's way of helping you deal with the situation so you can get help. Our psyche can do the same thing with emotional pain, but it functions in the opposite way: you feel the pain, but you don't see it because your mind numbs you to it. Still, it's there operating in the subconscious all the same. That unseen pain will manifest in the life choices you make *and don't make,* in how you get triggered, in the partners you choose, and in how you engage in your relationships. It manifests, but you don't see it specifically. You only see the fallout.

· · ·

Your partner sees the fallout of your unseen pain as well, as Lynnea pointed out when talking about the choices Eliza made while in college. Often, they can trace the way your pain manifests back to its source, identifying what it is that your mind shields you from seeing fully. They may be in a unique position to gently help you peel away the protective armor that keeps you from seeing, and thereby addressing, the stone that lies at the center of the ripples of pain that spread through your life. So now, when this question comes up, you are about to hear what your partner sees that you refuse to look at because you've been numbing that pain. As scary as that can be, remember that the pain is there whether you look at it or not. And if you look at it, you're one step closer to healing it.

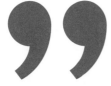

You can't erase someone else's pain, but you can fill it with love.

—DaiAwen

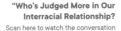

"Who's Judged More in Our Interracial Relationship?
Scan here to watch the conversation

It's possible that when your partner points out the pain you haven't been addressing, this will create more tension for you because they are pushing you to look at it. When this happens, it's not uncommon for one to feel like it's them that's the problem, that their effort to guide you toward—and therefore, through—your pain is something they are doing to hurt you instead of a service they are doing for you. Do your best to frame this offering of awareness as a gift, a gift they are giving to you to help you on your path to healing.

Suggestions for How to Process This Question

Slow down. Take a few long breaths. Usually, when we are in pain we speed up to get through it as soon as possible. Your instinct is fight or flight. But the trick is to stay in it. Know that your mind is doing its best to protect you. Tell yourself there is something to learn here and practice sitting with your pain. It will pass. Everything does. "This too shall pass" isn't just some great biblical line, but also a profound truth. A fundamental principle in life is that change is constant. Nothing remains the same. Ever.

Knowing that, don't rush your response to this question. By slowing down you'll be creating the space needed for healing. Don't deny yourself the opportunity to grow when pain or fear presents itself. Instead, slow down and thank it. Thank life for the opportunity to heal and grow.

• • •

The following process has impressed me when seeing participants work their way through the responses to this question:

First, take a few breaths to slow down.

Second, thank the other for sharing what they are experiencing. Being grateful for your partner articulating what they know could be very painful for you is a wonderful sign of their trust and faith in the connection of your relationship.

Third, sit with it. See what comes up and don't react. Just witness the feelings and thoughts that arise. There is no need to respond. You don't have to solve anything, defend anything, explain anything. Just be with it. Watch how it plays out in your psyche. Create that distance between you and the emotions you're having. Doing so will enable you to learn from them more easily.

Finally, if you'd like, play back what you heard your partner say. This is a really valuable experience because you are speaking about yourself but from their perspective. And that gives you a kind of out-of-body experience. More importantly it begins to separate the pain from who you are. You aren't the pain; you are just the person experiencing the pain. Often we forget that important distinction. We are so entwined with the pain that we believe the pain *is* us. It's not. It's just something we carry with us.

• • •

A question worth exploring is *How does the pain serve me?* Sometimes we carry the pain because it enables something else in us—a reason not to do something, or a justification for not pursuing something we really desire.

Allow yourself to ruminate on whatever comes up for the next few hours, or days even. Maybe something important will come out of that directly; maybe it will take more time, more conversations, more exploration. The point is, the seed of growth has sprouted and you have articulated the pain, brought it out of the shadows and into the light. Now you can see what it can bloom into.

What is one experience you wish we never had and why?

One person's internal wound can have a profound emotional effect on their partner. Even though it was caused by something that only one of you experienced directly, it can insinuate itself into the space between the two of you, becoming something of a shared cross that's borne by both partners. But what about painful experiences that involve both of you from the outset? What about the bumps in the road you've endured together?

Having addressed your individual wounds in Question 7 (*What is the pain in me you wish you could heal and why?*), Question 8 now asks you to look at a collective wound you share with your partner. Revisiting this uncomfortable experience can reinforce a strong bond of solidarity between you, invite a sigh of relief into your conversation as you discuss how this experience has come and gone, or, most crucially, allow each of you to get a new perspective on an event that you look back on as painful, perhaps allowing you to see it in a whole new light.

Exploring the Collective Wound

The main difference between what you discuss here and whatever sources of pain you explored in the previous question is that experiences that cause collective wounds affect your union; it is a pain that your connection holds. That's not to say that this experience was either of your faults or that either of you did something to cause it. Rather, by nature of it being a shared experience, it couldn't have happened the way it did without your relationship existing in the first place. It is yet another example of the uniqueness that your connection with your partner has brought into the world. Whether it's something beautiful or something painful, your relationship is a constant source of creation, a potent sun around which an entire galaxy—filled with wonder and woe and everything in between—revolves. As you and your partner respond to this question, can you find the blessing in that together?

Notice how the question order has put the individual wound and the collective wound in conversation with each other. Despite this key difference between a source of pain incurred individually and one experienced as a unit, asking these questions one after the other may illuminate a connection between the two. One of the patterns in life that can be most difficult to break is the way we relate to pain. How we interpret and how we decide to either engage with or push away the things that hurt us can become a part of our identity. Perhaps it became an unconscious way of moving through the world in our childhood and adolescence, which may not serve us any longer. Might exploring a collective wound with your partner and juxtaposing each of your reactions to it allow you to discover a pattern in the way you react to painful experiences?

As you and your partner respond to this question, it's a good idea to pay attention to where each of your subjective perceptions of the undesirable experiences in your past align and where they diverge. When asked in {THE AND}, either a couple will have exactly the same experience in mind and agree on what said experience means in the context of their relationship, or their responses might differ in interesting and illuminating ways. Maybe they pick different moments altogether, or maybe they pick the same moment but interpret it differently. One partner might see a collective wound as something they absolutely wish hadn't been a part of their experience, but the other might see it as a necessary rite of passage.

Returning veterans of many conversations for {THE AND} who presumably practice having these sorts of intimate conversations in their daily life, Ben and Sidra already had a big-picture perspective on a collective wound when this question came up for them. We can see how even the most undesirable experiences can become valued stepping stones on the way to a happy and healthy relationship. When Ben poses this question to Sidra, she's already looking at the painful moments in their past in this light. Before she responds, I feel like I can see her thinking back to those difficult experiences. Just from observing her expression, it seems to me like she's really dropping in, letting emotions she felt in the past wash over her once more in this moment. But even with those emotions having entered the space of their conversation, she speaks from her present perspective—a holistic viewpoint where she can see the entirety of her relationship with Ben spread before her.

"It's really hard to say that I wish X had never happened because it's the sum of the series that brings us to now," she says. "Could there have been easier ways of learning those lessons? I don't know. Sometimes you only get those lessons if you get your ass kicked. I easily could say that I wish we'd never moved to Pittsburgh." Ben nods, recalling this specific collective wound they shared. "I have never been so depressed," Sidra continues. "I've never been so sad. I've never been so lonely . . . I felt so adrift from myself . . . But I can't say I wish it didn't happen. Our relationship falling apart was what allowed us to rebuild a relationship that was stronger. It's hard to say I'm grateful for all of it, but I am. I'm grateful for where it's brought us."

Marcela & Rock: A Profound Reframing

One of my favorite things about {THE AND} is getting to watch participants make paradigm-shifting realizations in real time. What happens when Marcela asks Rock, her husband of seven years, what experience he wishes they'd never shared is a prime example of how having an intimate conversation can directly lead to a healing shift in perspective.

"My answer is one word," Rock says, lifting his eyebrows. "Prison."

"I'd say the same thing," Marcela replies, nodding her head. "Prison."

Here the couple has agreed—immediately and unequivocally—that this one experience is the greatest collective wound they share. But as their conversation develops, it becomes clear that they each

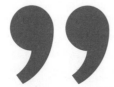

What I never want you to forget is the amount of light you have amidst the darkness you've been through.

—Raheem

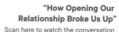

"How Opening Our Relationship Broke Us Up"
Scan here to watch the conversation

have very different interpretations of that wound and its meaning in their relationship.

"If I could change our relationship," Rock says, his long dreadlocks tied back neatly behind his head, "it would be a portion of our history." He looks down and the pace of his words slows. He seems to be reliving all the difficult situations that resulted from his incarceration. His voice sounds almost as if it's being stretched across time. "It was very complicated to make it through a lot of the situations that we've made it through."

The moment he finishes speaking, Marcela jumps into the conversation. "Yeah," she says, "but if we wouldn't have lived that, we wouldn't be here today, married for so long, and have the relationship we have." Here, she slows down, making sure that each of her words carries a certain weight. It looks to me like she desperately wants to offer them to Rock in order to absolve him of some of the residual pain he's been carrying for years. "We had to endure what we [endured] in the past. We had to be where we were at. We had to go through all we went through." Even as she relives these heavy moments in her mind, the brilliant, joyous smile she flashes many times throughout this conversation animates her eyes, finding ways to speak through her serious expression.

As she speaks, Rock's jaw has been slack. It looks to me like he's in nothing less than shock that his partner could see the many trying moments born of that huge word he dropped earlier—*prison*—as net positives. I can almost see the memories and emotions attached to them being shifted around inside his mind.

"All the things we have accomplished," Marcela goes on. "We have a son together. We wasn't supposed to have children. We wasn't supposed to have what we have now." It's clear to me that the subtext there is that she believes they wouldn't have grown as individuals and collectively had they not faced their challenges as they had. Doing so delivered many gifts beyond what either of them had ever expected.

Rock bites his lip. He leans back in his chair. It looks like he can't believe it. But then he looks up at the ceiling. He takes a deep breath, taking in this tectonic reframing of his and Marcela's history together. And he relaxes. It looks to me like he accepts it, like he sees their past, for the very first time, from the holistic perspective Marcela has just offered. He lifts his eyebrows again, looking impressed.

"That was a pretty profound answer right there," he says.

The Rack Focus Moment

It looks to me like Rock experienced something I like to call a "rack focus moment"—an instant of insight that brings the past suddenly and clearly into context in one's life. We use the term "rack focus" all the time when shooting films. When you're operating a camera on set, to rack focus means bringing a shot into focus. That same jolt of clarity can happen when we revisit moments from our past, especially while in conversation with a partner. Even though he's wearing dark glasses, you can see this happening to Rock as Marcela expresses nothing less than gratitude for the difficulties they shared. If you watch their full conversation, you'll see that these aren't trivial bumps in the road; Marcela is speaking with gratitude about years of a relationship maintained in spite of the barbed wire of death row, the locked doors of solitary confinement, and all the challenging moments that involves. The power of this sentiment has an immediate impact on Rock. In a flash, he sees the purpose of their shared suffering, sees how together they have turned it into their shared joy.

I know just how incredible feeling a shift like this can be. Filming {THE AND} gifted me a rack moment of my own. I've shared with you that for decades my parents' divorce and the subsequent struggles with allowing intimacy into my life were a source of pain for me. Failed relationships and instances of sheer frustration and despair litter my twenties and thirties like breadcrumbs, forming a path I stumbled down clumsily. I carried the torment of those experiences for so long. For years it seemed like nothing more than pointless suffering. But then, when I was about forty, filming one of the hundreds of conversations for {THE AND}, something opened up for me and my perspective on my past totally changed. I saw the clear arc of my life thus far, the way that all my suffering was the catalyst for this project that I love so dearly and which fulfills me more completely than I could have ever imagined.

All of that time spent honing my skill as a filmmaker, pursuing my passion, I was wondering why exactly I was doing it. But those conversations I witnessed showed me how focusing on human connection was my calling. All of those moments between participants in {THE AND} where a level of profound intimacy is reached, felt, and offered back and forth between two souls in a sacred dance of emotion was something I never witnessed or thought possible as a young person. None of that could have happened had I not experienced that painful initial wound and all the suffering that followed, because it created the hunger which created the gift that I can now share with others.

When all of that coalesced for me in one scintillating instant of clarity, I felt this huge weight lifted off of my shoulders. It hadn't all been for nothing. There had been a purpose to my pain and confusion. For so many years I'd had no idea what it was, but then, eventually, my rack focus moment hit me like a freight train and I almost felt myself get ripped apart by the force of my gratitude for the journey treaded.

● ● ●

That's my story. Now what's yours? Whatever it may be, it's playing out for you right now as you read these words. Is there a wound— individual or collective—that you carry, wondering as it stings what it could possibly be for? I truly believe that if you move through the world with an open heart and a curious mind, at some point you'll understand why things happened the way they did. Your rack focus moment will arrive. And you will have more than one such moment. You'll have many. Take it from a person who couldn't fathom having an intimate connection with another human being and who is now the author of a book about how to not just make intimate connections but how to further deepen them.

Suggestions for How to Process This Question

This can be a tough question where difficult experiences are relived or brought into a new light. Emotions will certainly come up. But emotions need to come up and be felt in order to be let go. Not thought about, but actually felt. Much like a photograph is worth a thousand words, an emotion is worth a thousand thoughts. So stop thinking and simply feel.

This is what people like to call processing their emotions. But what does processing emotions mean? That's a needlessly complicated way of saying it. We could just as easily say "feeling" our emotions instead. All emotions want is to be felt. It's when you try to resist emotions, try to mitigate the full force of them instead of feeling them or judge yourself for having them, that they stick with you. You'll find that if you really allow yourself to feel your emotions, they will go on their way much faster, cutting out those thousand thoughts in an instant of embodied feeling, and leave you to experience whatever new emotion life throws at you next. This question gives you and your partner a space to do that together.

Sometimes nothing even has to be said in response to this question. This happens all the time on {THE AND}. Both partners know what the collective wound is, but they don't want to talk about it on camera. However, in the most constructive conversations, they don't brush it off and move on when this happens. They sit in the emotion silently, making eye contact and dropping into their bodies. Sometimes that's all that's necessary.

And once you've done this—felt the emotion—let it go. Moving forward once you've taken the time to feel is key. You don't need to get stuck in a place of venting about something difficult. In the space you've created here for this conversation, let that pent-up emotion out. Let yourself feel it. Allow your partner to feel it. Recognize it, and then let it go. Once the emotion has been felt, you'll be able to work through the actual issue that caused it with greater clarity.

What do you think you are learning from me?

So far, no scientist, great philosopher, or wise spiritual leader has come up with a definitive answer we all agree on for why we're here on planet Earth. I don't profess to be any of those, but, taking into consideration what I've learned throughout the course of my life, if I had to give it my best guess, I'd say that we're here to learn—and no, not to learn the sort of esoteric knowledge that yogis seek when they meditate alone in caves; we're here to learn from each other. You can learn valuable, even profound lessons from your college professor, your coworker, or the guy who cuts you off in traffic. But the deepest lessons in life, the sacred lessons, are the ones you learn from the people you are closest to. Our intimate relationships and the people we build them with can be our greatest teachers.

So, what are you learning from the person sitting across from you? What enduring gifts have they offered up that you'll carry with you when you walk away from this conversation or from the relationship itself? What is the experience of engaging in a synergistic dance with another human being teaching you day in and day out?

Inviting in the Salve of Gratitude

This question comes right after a succession of opportunities to delve into discomfort and conflict that lead you into the conversation's cathartic climax. That part of the experience can sometimes feel like doing surgery on your relationship, cutting through all its defenses and exposing the vulnerable parts of you and your partner that lie intermingled beneath. Maybe deep-seated resentments were exhumed and brought into the light. Maybe painful memories were dug out so that they could be held together in a nurturing and supportive space. Or maybe not. No matter what came up for you and your partner, take a deep breath and a moment to acknowledge your courage for having come out the other side. Congratulations, that part of the conversation is over. You made it through. You survived—your relationship hopefully stronger, healthier, and revitalized for having elected to undergo this procedure. But you can't just leave the relationship lying there on the operating table. Now is the time to begin stitching it back up by inviting a direct appreciation for your partner and all that they'd offered you into the space.

There are valuable lessons to cherish that you are constantly learning from your partner, things that you can be grateful for no matter what has come up over the course of the last several questions. This is where the focus now shifts: to the irrevocable gifts your partner has given you just by being in your life. If your connection was challenged by the preceding questions, it is now reaffirmed as you are invited to appreciate it in a new light. Being vulnerable didn't kill you. In fact, what it did was bring you to a place of gratitude, where you can look at the cherished lessons your partner is teaching you.

Notice how this question asks your partner to share what they are learning from you, versus asking them to tell you what they are teaching you. This puts them in a place of admiration and acknowledgment rather than one of ego. By recognizing that they are learning, they speak from a place of humility. They show you ways in which they are the student and you the teacher. When the question is reversed and you have the opportunity to respond, that power dynamic flips; you become the student and they, the teacher. This push and pull highlights the symbiotic interplay you are both engaged in as you live a life together, one that is unique to your specific connection.

Andrew & Jerrold: Tailor-Made Mirrors

Let's revisit Andrew and Jerrold's conversation for a moment to see both the value of the learning our partners can offer us, as well as how the lessons they teach us tend to be unique and specific to the singular connection we share with them and them alone. Thus far, we've witnessed this married couple confront multiple points of conflict in their relationship in Questions 4 and 7. We've seen them bravely admit mistakes they've made and heard them share how they've turned those challenges into opportunities for real growth. Therefore, it's not surprising that when Jerrold asks Andrew what he's learned from him, the first word that comes to Andrew is "patience." But as he unpacks this single word in his deep, resonant voice, Andrew finds himself sharing lessons Jerrold taught him that have completely reoriented his perspective on life.

"You've been a living example of a person who has an unbelievable amount of patience in a way that I've never seen in anyone else," Andrew tells his husband. "A bomb could go off, people could be going completely out of control, and you'd be chill and fine and I'd be losing my shit. You're always just telling me to calm down. That it's going to be OK. That's why [at] the beginning of our relationship, for the first two years, I thought you were crazy."

At this, Jerrold laughs out loud, flashing a brilliant, playful smile and looking down toward his feet.

Andrew continues: "I was like, 'This guy is secretly fucked up and he just doesn't know it yet. And we're [eventually] going to have some breakdown and he's going to be like, *Oh my God, this is all a farce that I put on!* And it's not. It's totally real!"

Here Andrew starts to laugh a little too. He seems blown away by the fact that he used to believe genuine patience and calm were impossible attributes for a person to possess. Through his laughter he goes on to say, "It wasn't until I talked to my brother that he was like, 'Yeah, some people are actually emotionally healthy.' Some people . . . are actually good people."

By simply being himself, Jerrold was able to teach Andrew so much more than just how to slow down, be calmer, and how to practice patience. Seeing how Jerrold genuinely and honestly believed things would be all right and that he would willingly care for him in moments

"

You make me feel like I've done something good with life. I feel completed with you.

—Chris

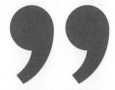

"We're So in Love, People Think We're Lying"
Scan here to watch the conversation

of stress, Andrew learned that people's behavior can be trusted and taken at face value, that kindness and patience aren't always just a façade. I can only imagine how this revelation has affected Andrew's interactions, not just with Jerrold, but with anyone he comes into contact with. Jerrold became a mirror for him, reflecting back at Andrew his own suspicion of people who seemed to be, as he put it, "emotionally healthy," as well as the places in which he, Andrew, could look to grow in order to reach the level of "emotional health" he saw in Jerrold.

But even this profound lesson was just the beginning of what Andrew says he learned from his husband. He shares that through their specific synergy, their unique and singular connection, Jerrold expanded his idea of what is possible in life.

"Given my background . . . my family and how religious and how repressive their ideology and theology was," Andrew continues, "I grew up in a world where I just never thought that I was going to be able to have certain things. I was never going to be able to get married to somebody without wondering whether I was making a mistake. I was never going to be able to be an authentic person. I had this whole life carved out for myself [with] all of these limitations of what my life would look like. And then since meeting you and having a relationship with you and marrying you, it's just surreal, because I just never thought that this would be a possibility for me, or that members of my family would come around and actually support us."

Before Jerrold came into his path, Andrew never could have believed that the life they share—married as two gay men—would have been an option for him considering his conservative upbringing. But to his surprise, that ended up being not just a possibility, but his day-to-day reality. Beyond that, he learned, to his utter shock, that his religious family could and would accept his marriage with another man. Andrew's perception of how the world worked, of what his life and future could hold, changed fundamentally because of his relationship with Jerrold. I find that in itself to be beautiful, incredible, and moving.

But I'd like to draw your attention to the next thing that Andrew tells his husband, as I find it to be one of the most important lessons to take from this couple's wonderful story. You see, Andrew doesn't believe that the paradigm shift he experienced could have happened with anyone else. It was Jerrold, and only Jerrold, who could have brought this expansion of his idea of the possible into his life, changing him and his outlook forever.

"A huge part of that is you," Andrew tells his partner. "It's not just that [my family] was like, 'Oh, I accept you now.' It's because of the person that *you* are. You are like the golden boy to bring home to people to whom you want to be like, 'You have a problem with our relationship? Meet this incredible person and then I dare you to talk shit about him. Now you have to really think critically about why you think relationships are or aren't morally correct.'"

It was Jerrold, and Andrew's specific synergy with him, that was able to open up both Andrew and his family to new possibilities. Could another person have done this for Andrew and his loved ones? Or are we and our partners like puzzle pieces, like tailor-made mirrors, making connections and reflecting back certain parts of us that no other person could in precisely the same way?

When anyone is in a truly intimate relationship, both they and their partner are in a unique position to impart certain lessons that only they can impart. So what is it that you're learning that only your partner could have taught you? You have already told them about the wonderful experiences they've gifted you, the quotidian moments of intimacy they bring into your days, the ways they might have hurt you, and the ways they have supported you as you've navigated your own pain. Here you can share with them the ways in which they've made you a better person, or, as in Andrew's case, have allowed you to step into new and more open ways of being in the world.

This is, of course, a gift they've given you. But it is also a service that they are doing for the entire world. By teaching you and thus helping you to grow, they are the catalyst for an infinite chain of more thoughtful interactions that you will carry out with everyone you meet. After any difficult moments they have just experienced in this conversation, isn't expressing your gratitude for the change they catalyzed in you a beautiful way of bringing your partner back into awareness of their unique and special power?

Suggestions for How to Process This Question

What if you are asked this question and feel like you have nothing nice to say about the things your partner is teaching you? Or what if it seems like they aren't teaching you anything at all?

If this is your gut reaction, don't worry. That's OK. But rather than let this apparent dearth of deep learning lead you into an emotional response based in judgment and pain, take a breath and try to clear the space. There is a lot of heaviness that the two of you have just moved together over the last several questions floating around, and it might be clouding your ability to look at your relationship through the lens of gratitude. Give that atmosphere the time it needs to dissipate so that you can see clearly. To do this, look deeply into your partner's pupils for at least ten seconds. Remember these are the eyes that are with you through thick and thin. These are the pupils that reflect *you* back to *yourself*. Take a few deep breaths and allow the gratitude for their presence to come into you. Treat it as a brief meditation, where your focus is on your breath and on new emotions that arise, rather than emotions that are reverberations of all the ground you two have just covered. If you do this, I can almost guarantee that you will find *some* positive lesson your partner is teaching you.

Feel free to get creative with your definition of "positive." Maybe your partner is teaching you that you would benefit from setting firmer boundaries, or that you want a partner who is an attentive listener, or the way that you specifically can grow from conflict in a healthy way. Or maybe the most positive thing that you've learned from them up to this point is that you want to have more of these kinds of conversations in your life, and you appreciate them participating in this conversation with you. Even if the lesson they're teaching you is that you don't want to put up with their shit anymore, thank them for it. That is still a precious gift which, in time, you will be grateful to them for bringing into your life.

What is one experience you can't wait for us to share and why?

If a shared past is the relationship's anchor, dreams of the future are the wind in its sails. You've come a long way in this conversation; both you and your partner have learned a lot about your connection and currently stand in the figurative crow's nest of your ship, with a bird's-eye view of your story together. This is a question that asks you both to look toward the horizon and imagine what lies beyond it. How do you see your lives unfolding together? What is it about tomorrow that fills you with excitement? And do those same things excite your partner? Do your dreams for the future align? What is it that's pulling you both into the next chapter of your shared story?

Identifying Mutual Dreams

You've experienced the grounding, intimacy, vulnerability, and healing of the preceding questions; now it's time to start looking ahead. Having steeped yourselves in both the beauty and the difficulties of your relationship, by the time you arrive at Question 10, where your relationship stands in the present moment should be clearer to you than it was before you began this conversation. Even if you feel more confused about your relationship than when you started, that itself is more information than you had when you first sat down to ask Question 1. Therefore, this is a perfect opportunity to explore what you hope will be next for both of you and an offering to consider why you are still in this relationship.

A shared history may be your foundation, but what kind of home are you hoping that foundation will support? Hopefully this conversation has seen you explore a great deal of the fruitful learning and growth you and your partner have provided each other in the past. But do you see the possibility of more learning, more growth in your future? Is there a mutual project—whether it's raising children, a shared business, or any sort of mutual goal—that you're actively working on, or planning to work on, together? And, crucially, does it excite you both? Does it hold enough of a draw that it makes dealing with the rocky waves of the present worthwhile?

This question harkens back to Question 1 (*What are your three favorite memories we share and why do you cherish them?*), where we explore what unique experiences you share due to your synergy. Here we are looking to the future for what new experiences your connection will create that excites you both. Hopefully, envisioning your dreams will provide both of you with a palpable sense of shared excitement. Answering this question is an opportunity to connect over the joys you have yet to experience and to open yourselves up to playful imagining. It can both be an invitation to share in the fun of planning and serve as a moment of reassurance. Imagining the things you can achieve, the places you can go, the life you can share—it can make any current challenge you've identified over the course of this conversation feel worth facing. Let this response hold the potential to propel you into the future together.

Or, let it show you how despite your shared history and cherished memories, you and your partner are on different trajectories. Are your aspirations things that excite both you and your partner, or do they just excite you? It's a good idea to really focus in on whether there are things that you want to achieve in the future, not just individually, but as a team. I'll never forget how once, when I was talking with one of my mentors—a wise, inquisitive soul, father of three, living in Berkeley with expansive life experience—he made the importance of sharing a collective dream with one's partner crystal clear. His youngest child had just gone off to college and he told me that now that their project of raising their three children was winding down and nearing completion, he and his wife had begun discussing what their next shared endeavor would be. If they couldn't think of one, he told me, they would consider going their separate ways, even after many years of marriage. Without something that they were building toward together, even if it weren't as concrete as raising children, they weren't sure there'd be enough in their relationship to keep them both feeling fulfilled for

"
I like the idea of us planning our futures together, to be back in the same place again.
I like knowing you're going to be there when I come home.
It makes me happy.

—Erica

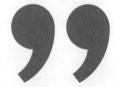

"Watch This Couple Propose"
Scan here to watch the conversation

years to come. Being in a relationship is the opportunity for mutual dreaming. Together. That's not to say you can't have your individual dream for yourself. However, it's a valuable exercise to ask yourselves what is the mutual dream that you can share, that lights both of you up, and that is only possible with both of your participation.

Keep in mind that turning those dreams into realities could require a lot of hard work and cooperation. This question gives you the space to examine the relationship while it's still laying there on the operating table, to look down at your ship from the crow's nest and see it holistically, considering all its strengths and all its blemishes that you've explored in the conversation until now. Have you and your partner identified some leaks in your ship? How do you feel about the severity of those leaks given where you want to go? Are you both charting the same course, or are your individual desires drawing you down divergent paths? As this question helps you both identify what it is that's pulling you forward into the future, this is a good opportunity to consider if the vessel you're in is fit to cover the distance between you and where you're going.

Ikeranda & Josette: A Light at the End of the Tunnel

We filmed the conversation between Ikeranda and Josette in 2020, while the entire world had a historic case of cabin fever thanks to the COVID-19 pandemic. When Ikeranda—a woman who carries herself with a confident, almost regal bearing, wearing pink lipstick and black-framed glasses—asks her partner, "What is one experience you can't wait for us to share and why?" Josette's eyes get a faraway look in them. It looks to me like the prototypical facial expression of the dreamer, of someone who has been able to fully step into the joy of imagination.

"There's a lot," Josette says happily, flashing a warm, calm smile from under her crown of silver braids. "There's so much we have—"

Ikeranda has been watching Josette's imaginings with a look of contentment, but she cuts her off, bringing her back to the present moment. "What is the thing that we talk about that we want to do as soon as the world opens up? With the family?"

"Oh!" Josette suddenly remembers. "Travel to Africa." She nods, I'd assume thinking back to the many conversations they've had about this future adventure. "I guess you're right. That's what I was going to say. There's so many things and we haven't done a lot of traveling together. We've traveled separately. So one of the biggest things I want to do—with the family, yes—but I just want to take off and see more of the world with you."

As those last words leave her lips, I can see full-blown, almost childlike, excitement creep into Josette's eyes. It's clear that this has been a dream of hers for many of their sixteen years of marriage. And the fact that it was Ikeranda who brought it up in the first place by alluding to past discussions that centered on their upcoming trip confirms that this is a dream that both partners share. As Josette finishes speaking, I feel like I can see Ikeranda's expression start to mirror her partner's. They both want this.

Watching these two talk with such excitement and hope about what they both want to do when restrictions lift and borders open, it seems clear to me that this shared dream must have been one of the things helping them get through the myriad difficulties of lockdown. Sometimes the power of a shared dream is so strong, it can be the light at the end of even the longest, darkest tunnels.

When Love Stops Being a Verb

Making a distinction between mutual dreams and individual dreams is extremely important. In multiple conversations they had for the {THE AND}, returning participants Keisha and Andrew each got the opportunity to ask each other this question. Even though the conversations were filmed years apart, they each answer their partner within seconds, authoritatively speaking the same answer. "A baby!" Keisha basically shouts, after Andrew has asked her this question. Then later, in a follow-up conversation, Andrew answers the same question with a matter-of-fact shrug: "Having kids." This is clearly the couple's shared dream—the thing they've envisioned through so many ups and downs, the thing pulling them into the future.

But what if you and your partner don't share the same dream? What if you want different things? What if you're willing to make some concessions to appease your partner's dream, but it doesn't really excite you, doesn't fill you with an eagerness to leap into your next chapter together? This might be the most common situation that gives rise to that feeling of, "I love you, but I'm not *in* love with you." You have grown, you have changed, and you still love your partner. But there isn't that excitement about a shared future anymore. Regardless of the lasting feeling of love you feel for each other, your respective passions in life are pulling you in different directions and therefore out of the active aspect, the verb form, of *being* in love.

This is an experience that I know intimately. In my early thirties, I'd been dating a partner whom I cared about very much. We were living together and I was even thinking about proposing to her. But at a certain point, about two and a half years into our relationship, things started to shift. There was a loss of energy, and the relationship was suffering from a drop in commitment from both of us that hadn't been there before. In an effort to sort all of this out, we went to see a couple's therapist. In one session, the therapist asked us about our dreams for the future. Without hesitating, I said that I wanted to have a home base from which I, my partner, and our future children would travel the world while I made films and worked on creative products. I wanted to live in South America for a year and, at some point, in Japan. I didn't want to be moving every two weeks, but I wanted my future to be filled with new experiences for me and my future family. As I was saying this, I felt a surge of energy, this physical sensation of excitement. I was animated, engaged. I was visualizing my dream. Then it was my partner's turn to answer. She said that her dream was to own a brownstone in Brooklyn, and to live a happy life with her family there, and I could see the same energy I'd felt animating her as she imagined herself living this very different future.

While she spoke about her dream, all the excitement I'd been filled with as I'd talked about South America and Japan left me. I felt de-energized. I loved this person, but that wasn't the future I wanted for myself. The therapist noticed this. To her credit, she got right to the point. Seeing that we both wanted, and wanted badly, very different things out of life, she leveled with us.

"So, the only question that remains is do you want to rip off the Band-Aid fast or slow?"

She was giving us two options: end the relationship immediately or fight a losing battle against what we truly wanted out of our lives in an effort to minimize the inevitable pain of separation.

In the long silence that followed her words, I felt all the air in the room go cold. As that silence dragged on, it slowly dawned on me that neither of us had spoken up to offer a third option. I think both of us realized that the therapist was right, that if we were being honest with ourselves, there really was nowhere else to go but our separate ways. I felt myself fill with an agonizing sense of acceptance. This was it. We'd shared so many happy moments and we'd shared this revelatory one. But how could we share a future that didn't excite us both equally? How could either of us make the other—a person we loved—suffer the pain of knowing they were living someone else's dream and not their own?

We left the therapist's office before the full hour was even up and headed to a place we liked to grab some lunch. Over the meal, we both cried. But we also laughed. We were crying because we each felt a beautiful chapter of our lives coming to an end. And we were laughing because we truly still enjoyed each other's company, still felt joy just being in each other's presence. There was also some relief in that laughter. Ripping the Band-Aid off was, and would be, painful, but I was so glad to know that I wasn't pulling her off her path in life and that I, similarly, wouldn't let an attachment—no matter how wonderful—pull me off course either. I think we both felt proud of our decision to go our own ways, to end on a good note rather than letting an aversion to pain or a fear of being alone drag us into a future where we were bound to end up resenting each other sooner or later. Even if we weren't exactly happy to be breaking up, we were at least happy about that.

Suggestions for How to Process This Question

As always, I encourage you to focus on your emotional response as this question plays out. Does the future you and your partner are talking about fill your stomach with excited butterflies or does it leave you feeling . . . nothing? Remember that if your dreams don't align, compromise is an option. But as you discuss that compromise or as you envision it, tap into your feelings again. What do you want to create together? Even if that means a bunch of lazy Sunday mornings drinking coffee while reading the newspaper. It doesn't have to be big. It's just good when it's aligned and mutual. Does it excite you? Does it affect you emotionally?

Whether the conversation that arises from this question is filled with collective dreams that are perfectly in sync, finds you examining individual dreams for places they can be brought together, or makes you realize that the biggest dreams you and your partner share aren't of some distant moment in the future but of the joys you can reap out of tomorrow, be patient and take it slow. The only sure thing about the future is that you can't predict it. Dreams change and so do people. Look at everything that comes out of this question with a gentle curiosity. It takes time to watch your dreams take shape or to witness what

QUESTION 10: What is one experience you
can't wait for us to share and why?

151

they change into. And you have every right to change your dreams at any moment. For many, once you have children, your dreams change and what you prioritize for yourself gets put on the back burner in favor of the priorities of your children. So you change. What you value changes and thus what pulls you into the future changes. That is fine and absolutely expected. That is OK. We are simply talking about the dreams you currently have from this vantage point in your life, right now. Let them be the compass by which you navigate, but don't sacrifice the present moment in order to rush into them.

Shared dreams and goals are some of the most unique fingerprints of any relationship. They represent the middle part of the Venn diagram you and your partner create by being in each other's lives. Acting from that unique place of unity—literally making that place where you overlap into an action, into something you do together—is as sure a way as any to invite a deeper level of intimacy into your connection.

If this was our last conversation, what would you never want me to forget?

The penultimate question in your conversation asks you to project even further forward into the future, to the inevitable moment of separation that you and your partner will one day face. Whether it's the end of the relationship or the end of life itself that causes that separation, one day it will happen. Every story ends. And once a story is truly over, the door is closed on your ability to verbally express to your partner that most important aspect of the bond you shared. If you wait too long, you'll lose the chance to say anything you might have left unsaid. But what happens if you don't wait at all? If you choose to share those profound words in this very moment? Answering this question will show you that by choosing to speak up now, you don't lose anything. In fact, by doing so you stand to gain and to offer something extremely precious.

Reflecting Each Other's Light

Now that the conversation has carried through healing, reconciliation, and acknowledgment of what your partner has offered you on your journey together, this question asks you to sit in the awareness of that journey's end. Perhaps, given what has arisen in this conversation, you've decided that the end is imminent. Or maybe this experience has made you realize that you hope your journey together will continue on forever. If you're in the latter camp, I hate to be the bearer of bad news, but there's no such thing as forever. The energy that gives us and the entire universe we inhabit shape is, by nature, in a constant state of flux. Nothing lasts forever, and trying to force it to do so is a negation of life's inherent rhythm. The more you can embrace the ebb and flow implicit in all things—good and bad—the more you'll be able to let the tides of experience move through you with peace, grace, and awareness.

Whether your journey together ends tomorrow or fifty years from now, if you take a minute to imagine that future moment of separation from your partner, surely there are some final, important words you'd wish to impart to them. They could be words of advice, words of admiration, or just a pure expression of love. Try to conjure up those words now. How does it feel to envision yourself saying them out loud? Does it feel embarrassing? Cathartic? Scary? Overwhelming? Joyful? No matter what it is that you'd never want them to forget, right now—with that moment of parting still in the hazy distance—there's a good chance that your words seem too unwieldy, too big, or too heavy, to share with your partner knowing that you'll face them again tomorrow. That's why you're saving them for your last meeting. You're protecting yourself from having to experience the vulnerability that exposing the sheer power of your emotions would precipitate. But look at how far you've come just in the course of this conversation. By the time you reach this question, you'll have navigated powerful emotions and spoken from a place of vulnerability again and again. Therefore, the purpose of this question is to leverage the comfort and trust you've been building with yourself and with your partner, allowing you to take this golden opportunity to voice things that are so profound, so honest, so vulnerable, and so deeply rooted in your connection with your partner that you wouldn't say them under normal circumstances.

Of all the things I've learned during my time on this planet, few feel as true to me as the idea that the heart is made to love. That's all it wants to do. But over the course of our lives, certain experiences, as well as exposure to our culture, cause calluses to form over our hearts, blocking that outflow of love. This happens to almost every one of us; it's a natural part of being alive in this day and age. Rejection, abuse, and trauma all create internal scar tissue inside us, which attempts to act as a shield, protecting us from further hurt. Combine that with the rules that society teaches us about what's permissible to share, what level of emotion is appropriate in a given situation, and just generally how we're supposed to act in front of others, and you're left with an obstacle course of impediments for the pure expression of our love to navigate on its way out into the world. Thus, we often feel uncomfortable sharing the undiluted, undulled brilliance of the love our hearts naturally create. Instead of effortless, it feels difficult. We feel like doing so is cheesy or clichéd. But those feelings aren't really ours. They are the judgments of our culture that we've assimilated unconsciously and the discomfort we feel when emotion squeezes its way through all of that scar tissue we've accumulated.

The way to subvert those cultural judgments is to become aware of them, to realize that they are not yours, and to bravely speak from your heart when you feel moved to. Given the strength of our societal conditioning, that's not easy. So let this question be a gentle first step into bringing this practice more actively into your life. As we saw with the concept of "sacrifice" in Question 6 (*What is a sacrifice you feel you've made that I haven't acknowledged and why do you think that is?*), feel free to hide a little behind the fact that it is the question itself that's asking you to share something that might seem "cheesy." You can blame it on me if you like. Whatever it takes, committing to doing so in the context of this guided conversation will allow you to see just how much of a relief it is to let your heart really speak its truth. This is the time to do it. The level of trust you and your partner have built by moving through all the preceding questions together has created a space that's suited to this level of intimacy. Having tilled the land of your relationship, your connection, and your history together, you've earned this moment. Spoken in a space like the one you've cultivated, your partner is more likely to respond with deep gratitude than being put off or overwhelmed. You can't know just how much your honest words might mean to them.

• • •

When I think about what we can be for each other and the ways in which we can enrich each other's lives, I always come back to this quote from author and psychiatrist David S. Viscott: "The purpose of life is to find your gift. The work of life is to develop it. The meaning of life is to give it away." How many of us spend our time searching for gifts we already possess but aren't aware of? How many of us fumble through our lives unable to see our own beauty, our own wisdom, our

"

I love you in this world and all the worlds to come.

—Victoria

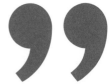

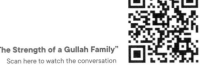

"The Strength of a Gullah Family"
Scan here to watch the conversation

own genius? The people closest to us can be powerful mirrors, reflecting that which we cannot see back at us. We've already seen this work in the context of partners helping each other notice, and thereby grow into a fuller expression of ourselves. But the same thing can happen with the best qualities we already have. Sometimes it takes someone in our life having the bravery to verbalize the full splendor of who we are before we become aware enough of our own brilliance that we can actively and consciously give it back to the world.

In 2008 I was filming a documentary of mine called *Americana*, a project that took me from Cuba to Mexico to Turkey, Albania, Vietnam, and Japan, as well as many other countries around the world as I searched for a global perspective on the question *What does it mean to be an American?* I found myself in Hiroshima, Japan, interviewing a survivor of the nuclear attack the city suffered on August 6, 1945. Having lived through so much, he had a lot of wisdom to offer. One of the things he said that stuck with me is that you only really get to know about a thousand people in your life. Over the course of an entire lifetime, that's not that many. What is the lesson that each of those few souls you come in contact with will offer you? What do you offer them? What kind of a mirror are you being for the people in your life? Unlike a literal mirror, we humans get to choose what it is we reflect back to the world and the people in it. What is it you're reflecting? How bright is the light you choose to shine back on your loved ones?

Kelly & Virgie: An Honest Answer

I'll never forget watching Kelly, a forty-four-year-old woman, ask her mother Virgie—in her eighties with silver hair and glasses—this question for {THE AND}. Immediately after she asks it, Kelly thinks she knows what her mother is going to say.

"Go to church?" she suggests, assuming, with a touch of knowing sarcasm, that her mother is going to take this opportunity to offer her moralistic advice. After over four decades of being Virgie's daughter, she's not exactly wrong.

"Yeah, keep your faith in God," Virgie replies, "and be kind to people. Because you're not the only human on the planet. Right?"

"That's news to me," Kelly says, laughing, the sardonic sense of humor the two women share now on full display.

After their shared laughter dies down, Kelly's face falls a bit. "Well," she says, "we're all out of questions." Is she a little disappointed? Does she instinctively feel something is missing? It looks to me like she is accepting that her mother just gave her a humorous response that, while true, doesn't exactly express the deep truth of their connection.

And then, Virgie comes into her own. She sets her shield of humor aside and speaks to her daughter directly from her heart.

"Well, there're many questions left in life," she begins, the flicker of a smile shining in her eyes, "but they'll just kind of tumble out occasionally. So, you feel free to always come to me. I may not give you the answer you want, but I will give you an honest answer."

"That's for sure," Kelly cuts in, clearly thinking that their conversation is going to continue having a quality of banter. But Virgie's tone changes, her voice deepening, coming from another place in her body. Kelly isn't expecting what comes next.

"And I will love you until the day I leave this earth," Virgie continues. "And then I'm going to have trouble communicating with you. But someplace up there, you'll know that I'm watching." A genuine grin of pride and love spreads over her face. "And I love you dearly. And you've brought so much to my life." Then, her smile fades, and suddenly as serious as she's been throughout the entire conversation, Virgie tells her daughter, "If I left this earth tomorrow, I will have had a full life because of you. You're my special baby."

And there it is. The pure, unadulterated truth of Virgie's heart, right there for Kelly to feel. If you watch how the pair sit together in the wake of that statement, it's clear that the depth of their profound connection has been expressed in words. Teary-eyed, they just look at

QUESTION 11: If this was our last conversation, what would you never want me to forget?

159

each other, taking in the moment. Judging by the look on Kelly's face, there's no doubting what a gift that was for her.

But Kelly didn't feel the full power of that gift until years later. Six years after we filmed their conversation, I received this email from Kelly's husband:

• • •

I wanted to reach out and let you know that Kelly's mom, Virgie, passed away last week at our home. It's been a rough few months but I have to tell you . . . today Kelly remembered {THE AND} experience she did with Virgie. She hasn't stopped watching the video today. I remember encouraging them to do that, and I'm so glad we have this document of their conversation.

So #1—thank you for creating this amazing collective narrative that allows my grieving wife to gain some solace in watching that conversation. Seriously . . . thank you.

As Kelly grieved the loss of her mother, she went back to that moment again and again, finding solace in the pure honesty and love conveyed in their conversation. What greater gift could we give each other than a truth that stretches beyond even the ultimate ending?

Make the End Now

Not long after filming *Americana*, I found myself working on Meghan L. O'Hara's acclaimed cancer documentary *The C Word*. As we filmed the movie, I had the honor and privilege of getting to know the late French neuroscientist and cancer revolutionary Dr. David Servan-Schreiber. David was a cancer survivor when I met him and had subsequently become a prominent figure in cancer treatment and prevention. But sadly, twenty years after his initial diagnosis, his cancer returned.

Before his passing, David wrote the book *Not the Last Goodbye: Life, Death, Healing, and Cancer,* dictating his prose in little more than a whisper during the last months of his life. It's a book filled with valuable information and learned wisdom, but the main thing I took away from it was David's crucial advice not to wait for the end to do what you want to do or to say what you need to say; better to make the end now.

The end rarely ever comes at a convenient moment. To wait for it to do so is a very risky gamble, one that isn't worth making, especially considering the only thing you risk by making the end now is your own emotional vulnerability. If you wait for life to present you with just the right moment to share your heart with your loved ones, you might miss out on an emotional exchange that will one day be permanently out of reach. So what are you waiting for? Make the end now. Speak the truth to your partner. Step into this moment that you've earned.

I myself have been guilty of waiting for the "right" moment to tell people in my life just how important they are to me and, unfortunately, suffered the heavy cost of not having made the end now. I was writing at a café in Brooklyn in April 2011 when I got the news: my close friend Tim Hetherington, a British photojournalist who only two months prior was on the red carpet at the Oscars nominated for Best Documentary for his film *Restrepo,* was killed by shrapnel from a mortar shell while covering the Libyan Civil War. For a moment, I just sat there in absolute shock. My vision blurred, and when it came back into focus on the screen in front of me, I saw the half-finished script for the film I'd been working on with Tim. I'd just been thinking about him, had been writing the project we'd spent hours discussing when I took a break, checked my phone, and saw that I had tons of missed calls and unread texts from his fiancée.

Whenever you see your screen filled with that kind of firestorm of messages, you know it's not going to be good news. I tried to prepare myself, but when I called her back and she told me what had happened, I felt my heart suddenly and completely break. I began to wrack my brain, trying to remember the last time I talked to him, the last thing we said to each other. I raced through memories of moments and conversations we shared. I looked through my phone for a voice mail from Tim just to hear his voice, but there weren't any. As I sat there in that café, my mind was flooded with all the things I wished I'd said to Tim. But all I could do was sit there, silently mourning my friend, those words spiraling around in my skull, unsaid. I realized our friendship was now a thread that would never grow further, but rather slowly wither away over time, living only in memory.

As terrible of an experience as that was, it solidified the idea of making the end now for me. It's something that I've since been sure to turn into a practice. You can express everything you'd want to express in that final moment many times over throughout your life. You can say goodbye many times over. You can say I love you many times over. You can say what's really important many, many times over. You don't need to wait until the end. And you shouldn't. The end rarely ever announces itself. It just happens. And at that point, it's too late. Don't feel like you need to wait for something special or something traumatic, because there might not be time to say the things that trauma moves you to say. What kind of world would we live in if we all made the end now, if we all spoke the deep truths of our relationships, if we became the mirrors our loved ones deserve?

Suggestions for How to Process This Question

Often, we don't think it's necessary to verbalize our most profound feelings about our partners. We think that it's just enough that we know what they are. If we choose to express them, we express them in nonverbal ways—in actions or smiles or touches or gestures that we hope convey these powerful emotions. And much of the time, this works; we do successfully transfer the depth of our love to our partner without a single word having to be spoken.

But think about it: we have the means to express those feelings in words, so why not do it? We may not have to say them, but why not render our emotions into words all the same? The most talented artist in the world might not have to keep painting once she's created something that's considered a masterpiece. But she has the ability to do so, so she keeps on giving her gift to the world. You have the ability to give your partner the gift of hearing the depth of your appreciation for them spoken in words. Why not make that choice? If we do come into close contact with only a thousand people in our lifetime, why not send a thousand ripples of honesty and connection flowing through humanity?

This quote by the Austrian philosopher Ludwig Wittgenstein sticks out to me from my days of studying philosophy at Oxford: "The limits of my language mean the limits of my world." For Wittgenstein, language was the limit of our understanding of the human experience. The more nuanced and complete our articulation of that experience, the richer it can become. Your words have power. Speak them and your world and that of those close to you will only become more vibrant.

QUESTION 11: If this was our last conversation, what would you never want me to forget?

163

Why do you love me?

How often do we ask this question in our day-to-day lives? Although its answer lies at the core of every moment, every interaction you share with your partner, rarely is it ever verbalized and put into specifics. When you love someone, you carry the certainty that your love for them exists deep within you. But do you ever stop to inspect it? You know it's there, but what does it look like? What does it feel like?

You may find that if you keep asking this question, peeling back layer after layer of intimacy, beneath them all lies nothing more and nothing less than an inarticulable feeling of closeness. The final gifts this conversation offers you are: one, the opportunity to articulate the reasons and nuanced feelings behind your love for your partner so that both of you are made aware of the specific divinity inherent in your connection; and two, the space to simply sit in silent awareness and awe of that transcendent force we call love.

A Transcendent Message

Of all the questions you have asked each other, this one can feel like the biggest. The conversation you've nearly completed has made you aware of the depth and complexity of your connection with your partner. Now I ask you to do your best to distill that universe of memories, feelings, challenges, pain, resilience, and sacredness into words. While filming {THE AND}, after this question was asked, I would often watch as the enormity of their love floods over the respondent before they attempted to articulate the summation of their feelings to their partner. It's definitely not an easy task. So if you find yourself feeling more challenged by this question than any of those that preceded it, don't worry; you're in good company. But remember, the preceding 11 questions have given you a good amount of practice with emotional articulation and speaking from a place of honest connection. As big as this question may seem, try your best to express the reasons why you love your partner. Doing so can be invaluable to them on so many levels.

I feel that giving your partner the gift of showing them why you love them has a level of importance that transcends your conversation, your relationship, and even what we consider "life" itself. It is my heartfelt belief that we come to this planet to learn from each other. We are all souls that have chosen to break away from the infinite in pursuit of a kind of knowledge that is only available in a finite existence. Much of that knowledge is gained from the loving connections we make with other souls on that same journey of discovery, the roughly thousand human beings referenced earlier by the Hiroshima survivor interviewed in my documentary. The simple act of looking into another person's eyes that you may have practiced at the beginning of this conversation is equivalent to glimpsing that infinite place we all come from and will return to—a place that is so comprehensively made of love it is impossible for our souls to even identify what love is while there. They need to come to a place where love is special, precious, and often contrasted by the disconnection of our world in order to be able to experience it. Therefore, explaining to our partner what it is that makes us love them allows that infinite part of them to get that much closer to completing its mission on Earth. Rising to the challenge of answering this question honestly is one of the most profound acts of service we can engage in.

What We All Really Want to Hear

Despite the power its answer can hold, it's so rare that we ever ask our partner, or even ourselves, this question. If it comes up at all, it's usually in the context of a fight or a breakup, when we're already smarting from some sort of hurt and looking at the relationship through that lens. Then, the question has an element of *Why am I so invested in this*

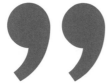

There is no end to why I love you.

—Ichak

"Will You Fall Apart if I Die?"
Scan here to watch the conversation

relationship? or *What am I getting from it?* as we try to rationalize the pain we are feeling.

This is why creating an intentional space in which to ask these questions is so important. Without having created a framework in which questions like this one can be asked and taken at face value, it would be difficult to really get an undiluted answer. But asking it now, at the end of a conversation in which your connection has been viewed from all angles and you have spent a good amount of time exploring it in a safe space that has allowed you both the freedom to feel emotionally vulnerable, you have the opportunity to really hear the reasons that your partner loves you, right now and in this very moment. Those reasons come from a place of seeing the relationship as a whole, with clear eyes and an open heart. At the end of the day, isn't this what you both want to hear most?

Let's return briefly to Rock and Marcela's conversation, the couple who'd maintained their relationship despite the challenges presented by years of incarceration, whose conversation we touched on in Question 8 (*What is one experience you wish we never had and why?*), to see how this holistic perspective can allow unique and impactful answers to blossom out of this question. When Rock poses it to Marcela, her eyes widen and she lets out a tremulous sigh as the power of her love for Rock hits her with full force. It doesn't take her long to condense those expansive feelings into a diamond of truth: "You make me whole," she says. "You make me a better woman."

Rock lets that sink in for a moment before he takes his turn answering. "Why do I love you?" he begins. "After eighteen-and-a-half years of [being] in and out of prison, I'm thirty-six, about to be thirty-seven. Everything that I've ever thought about having in my life from the very first time I was incarcerated at thirteen." He takes a deep, reflective breath and then exhales. "I [now] have everything that I've ever desired in life. You've assisted me with accomplishing everything that I knew I needed in my life so that I wouldn't go back to prison, so that I wouldn't be involved in the streets."

"So, I make you better?" Marcela asks with a wry smile.

"You've perfected my understanding of righteousness," Rock replies, and you can see in Marcela's eyes the relief and sense of pride, power, and understanding that statement gifts her after everything they've been through together.

Suggestions for How to Process This Question

It's not uncommon that when asked this question, participants' knee-jerk response is: "I just do." Sometimes that reaction can be another one of those cultural mantras rearing its head. We are taught that love is just . . . love. It's just a feeling, too mysterious, all-encompassing, and unconditional to ever put into words. I never understood truly unconditional love until my son was born. With my son, my love isn't a choice. It's something that nothing could ever take away from me or alter.

But we all choose to love our partners. And there's a special beauty in that. Think about what it is that causes you to make that choice and you'll be able to answer this question in a way that's true to you specifically, without just reciting a cultural mantra. As we've seen with Rock and Marcela, describing the seemingly indescribable with words is possible. However, it isn't always possible, or even necessary. Underneath the words you can or can't find to express your love, there's just pure feeling, and that, no matter how completely you master the skill of emotional articulation, is impossible to put into words. The only way to express it is through a deep, connective moment of silence, one in which that feeling is present and shining in your heart. The words that bracket this moment might be that very same "I just do." But if you truly drop into your emotions, if you call that feeling of love into the room and let it sit there with you and your partner, "I just do" will not be a cultural mantra; it will be an honest expression of your truth and, believe me, both of you will be able to feel that difference.

I'd like to leave you with one such moment that took place between Rafa and Douglas, the first couple we met in the early pages of this book.

"Why do you love me?" Rafa asks.

Before he answers this question, Douglas takes a moment to let his feelings for Rafa come to the surface. He nods his head a few times, connecting with them. Having explored those feelings so fully in their conversation up to this point, they're close at hand, and it only takes him a moment to let them sink in.

Douglas answers, "There's not a reason or a thing. And this is why it's so valuable. It's just—I just do . . . It just *is*. I love you and it's profound . . . It's just because."

Had they been spoken by another person, one who hadn't taken that key moment to drop into their feelings before speaking, those very same words could have been a cultural mantra. There is no way textually to show you the difference. But if you watch their conversation, if you see the truth glimmering in Douglas's eyes, the tears that fall from Rafa's in that sacred moment of connective silence that ends their conversation, you'll see exactly what I mean.

The two of them sit there for a long beat, not speaking, but simply staring into each other's black onyx pupils. Physically, the exact same thing that happened when they first sat down to have their conversation is happening again: they sit in silence, staring into each other's eyes. But this silence is different. Something—invisible but undeniably real—has changed, grown, strengthened. As they look into their partner's pupils, what do they see there? The infinite? The reflection of their own souls in another? Or simply the loving gaze of the person whom they've chosen to share the beauty of true intimacy with?

They stare into each other's eyes for a long while.

And then, simultaneously ending their conversation and beginning the next chapter of their relationship, Rafa whispers to his husband, "Ditto."

III: Before You Begin

You've seen how the power of questions can shape your possibilities, the components of what makes a powerful question, and how creating a safe space is imperative to a connective conversation.

But what happens when, during the conversation, things seem to go off the rails? What can you do to get it back on track? How is it best to engage with these 12 questions, or anytime you step into the space between? Here are some strategies for how to manage these kinds of challenges.

TROUBLESHOOTING: HOW TO COURSE-CORRECT

Having a deep and honest conversation can be a challenge, especially if you and your partner don't have much practice doing so. Putting these methods into practice will go a long way toward smoothing out any bumps in the road you may hit while traveling through an intimate discussion. But if you still find yourself struggling for any reason or are feeling nervous about getting started, that's OK. Here are some ways to easily diffuse the most common issues and concerns that might arise from this guided conversation, as well as tips for getting it back on track if you and your partner ever find yourselves stuck.

General Guidelines

Don't Come To This Conversation with Expectations or an Agenda

The goal of this conversation is for it to happen, nothing more. It doesn't need to change your life, it doesn't need to feel profound, and, most importantly, it doesn't need to solve anything. There's a chance that it will do all of those things and more, but coming to the conversation with an end result in mind is a sure way to doom it from the start.

If you've made it this far, the idea of having a conversation that will help you connect to your partner on a profound and intimate level may give you some sort of an emotional response. Maybe it feels interesting or exciting or like a challenge you feel will lead you to a deeper understanding of yourself, your partner, and your relationship. Possibly even to a more conscious way of being in the world? Even better. But I'd also hazard a guess that just after that emotional response arises out of your heart, your brain starts getting ideas and excitedly whispering them to you, possibly drowning out those heartfelt emotions. *What can you get out of this conversation?* your brain asks. And so, perhaps you started thinking about how this conversation could concretely make your relationship better, the specific things it might change in the way you and your partner interact. Could it fix that one issue that keeps coming up between the two of you, that one point of friction that always leads to a fight? Or perhaps you begin to fantasize about what a life-changing, powerful experience this conversation might be for you, how it could become a memory that you and your partner will cherish for years to come.

This is all normal. I wouldn't ever fault you for having thoughts like those, and if they provide you with the requisite motivation for deciding to actually go ahead and have the conversation outlined in this book, that's wonderful. However, once you have made that decision, it is of the utmost importance that you let those thoughts go. By the time you sit down to have this conversation, those thought-driven, result-oriented, head-generated motivations should be the furthest thing from your space. Let go of expectations. Focus instead on what led you here in the first place: that initial emotional spark of interest and curiosity around *just having the conversation* that bloomed from your heart.

You and your partner are not coming to this conversation so that two *brains* can connect. You are coming to it so that two *beings* can connect. Your brain gets to speak enough in your day-to-day conversations. This conversation is an opportunity for your heart to take center stage and fully say its piece. Once you've begun to engage with the questions, rely on deep listening—dropping in to your body and trusting those intuitive feelings before formulating your response to a question—as much as possible to ensure that the conversation stays guided by what your heart wants moment to moment, rather than by a rigid agenda that your head has prescribed. The mind is built to protect. The heart is built to connect. This is an opportunity to train yourself in letting your heart be heard. Stepping into this experience with an agenda won't allow that to happen. It will cause you to think rather than feel and to speak the careful, calculating discourse of the mind.

Honor the Sequence of These 12 Questions

I sincerely hope that the conversation this book guides you through is the first of many intimate conversations composed of thoughtful, powerful questions that you have in your life. Every one of them will be different. Maybe you'll make it a practice to play {THE AND} Card Game or the {THE AND} app. Maybe you and your partner will become so good at creating better questions on your own that you'll drop into these kinds of conversations without any sort of guidance whatsoever.

But for the specific conversation outlined in this book, I strongly suggest you do not ask these questions randomly. These 12 questions are sequenced in a very intentional way. As you have already seen, they aim to build a foundation of intimacy and connection by drawing on the past before moving into the joys and challenges of the present. Once those have been explored, the questions then ask you to look toward the future with a holistic view of the relationship fresh in your mind, before closing again on a note of pure connectivity.

Therefore, it's best to have this entire conversation in one sitting in order to experience each of these important beats on your journey to deeper intimacy. Choosing certain questions to ask at different times, especially if you haven't established what you are doing with your partner and created a safe space first, can potentially cause problems. But honoring the order of the questions outlined in this book ensures that you are prepped for any emotional distress you might find your relationship undergoing and creates the space for it to get the proper aftercare as well.

If at any point one or both of you feels like your conversation has led you to a place that's particularly heavy or dark, I encourage you to gently continue onward through these questions. Rest assured that they have been carefully designed to lead you out of the woods and back home. Keep moving forward—intentionally, compassionately, empathetically, slowly—and you'll get there together.

Remember to Slow Down

Make sure you and your partner have allotted enough time for this conversation so that you don't feel rushed and have the freedom to move through it as slowly as necessary. Rushing from question to question will encourage surface-level responses and will not allow time for deep, sometimes unexpected, discussions to bloom out of each question. The tangential discussions your answers can lead you to are often far more important than any direct answer.

Remember, the whole ethos here is to stop focusing so much on answers. So don't simply fire off an answer to a question and move on if there is a larger piece of the puzzle that you or your partner's response has started to unearth. Dig as deep as you need. Take the time to get your hands dirty. Let the conversation go where it wants and allow any guidance to come from your body. Let new questions arise out of the responses to these 12 questions. Just keep in mind that not all questions are equal, so do your best to be conscientious of how you construct any follow-ups. Ask and answer them completely, holistically, making space for the dance of deep listening and emotional articulation to play out at its own pace. Take your time.

What to Do if the Conversation Becomes Too Painful

While it's always important to move through this conversation slowly, this is especially true when the emotional tenor of the conversation spikes or if things become heated. When pain presents itself or conflict arises, there is a natural urge to speed up and try to rush out of pain and toward comfort, or to say your piece as fast as possible. Be aware of these traps, take a deep breath, and slow down in order to subvert them.

If there comes a time when you feel the natural urge to run away from the vulnerable place in which you've found yourself, try to remember what we learned in Question 7: *What is the pain in me you wish you could heal and why?* The safe and supported exploration of pain is what leads to healing. Pain ignored still hurts. And while treating any kind of pain is rarely comfortable, it is the only way for us to actually be free of it and move on. So sit together with the emotional pain. It's in the healing of the pain where our joy can deepen. Invite it in for a cup of tea. Let it say its piece and then move on to the next question, knowing that the 12 questions will naturally guide you back to more pleasant emotions soon enough.

Creative Listening

If you find yourselves in conflict, and you can feel yourself heating up and speeding up, I have two tools for you to consider that will help tremendously. One is called creative listening, a term coined by my good friend and software development leader Richard Tripp. Incredibly articulate and with a tenaciously creative mind, Tripp has played key roles in pioneering techniques for improving communication between software developers and business leaders (groups that are often in natural states of conflict). Creative listening, as taught by Tripp, is a simple and reliable way to shift the energy of the conversation toward building shared purpose through listening to one another not to respond, and not even to understand, but to help each other with the articulation of a new realization happening in real time.

Here is how it works: To ensure that you are actually listening to the other person, and for that speaker to know this, before you make any response, the first thing to do is to repeat what you understand the speaker to have said. You can begin with "To play it back" or "What I understand you to be saying is." This way the speaker knows that you are listening and attempting to understand, which is a refreshing alternative to the more common "listening to respond" that we often use as a default in our communication. Often we find ourselves fighting not because we want to be right or wrong, but rather simply from a desire to be heard. So when the speaker concludes their point, before you respond, repeat back to them what you heard.

Now they have three options. One is to say, "Yes, that is what I said." But what has happened here is that psychologically the speaker has relaxed because they know they've been heard. You just played it back to them and they know that you understand them. So the feeling as your conversation progresses is that we are on the same team and the same page, and we are sorting this out.

The second option for the speaker is to say, "No, that's not what I mean." How many times have you found yourself in a conversation where the listener jumps in and says, "It's like this," or tries to expand on what you're saying and it is not at all what you are saying. And yet, cultural norms tell us to say, "Yeah, kind of" and continue, instead of disagreeing with them, stopping, and clarifying. I've done this myself, especially when I was younger. But this is a very important intersection. Having the listener play back what they are hearing ensures that they understand you and the point you are trying to make. You can think of creative listening as a type of verbal processing where, instead of advocating to each other, we are assisting each other in articulating a realization happening in real time. So you keep this back-and-forth process going, the speaker making their point and the listener playing it back until the speaker feels that indeed their point of view has been heard. This doesn't mean you are agreeing with each other. It just means you are making sure that the conversation is proceeding in a space where shared understanding is a major priority, and each participant has the ability to state and evolve their point of view until they feel their realization has been clearly expressed and understood. Try this and you'll be amazed at how your body reacts when it knows it's been heard.

So you go back and forth until the speaker says, "Yes, that's what I mean," or a third option arises. Once the speaker has heard their words played back to them, they are seeing whatever it is they've said from a new vantage point. They hear it repeated back with new words, perhaps with more distinctions or nuances that they didn't originally articulate. They now have the full right to say, "Yes, that's what I said, but now that I hear it played back, I realize I don't believe it anymore." This happens more often than we like to admit. Hearing our own idea through another person allows us to disidentify from the idea enough such that we can evaluate it more deliberately than when we're trying to explain it ourselves.

When we don't feel heard, we close up and begin to conflate our desire to be heard with a desire to be right. But once you're heard, the space opens for you to look at your argument and see if it still holds, and even to possibly change your position after having heard your argument played back to you. Creating the space for this is what creative listening does. At work in The Skin Deep and with my partner at home, whenever I feel myself tighten up and want to control things, speed up, or head to conflict, I quickly utilize creative listening.

Implement Hard Rules

This is a small, albeit powerful tool that my father, Dr. Ichak Adizes, a pioneer in change management, uses in his methodology and practice of scaling cultural change. Being his sons, my brother and I got a lot of this when arguments were deteriorating. One of us would yell "Hard rules!" and we would all abide. Hard rules is an extremely helpful tool to immediately put a brake on things and to create the space for everyone to be heard in their entirety. After all, it's very difficult to get anywhere if you're cutting one another off and raising your voice to be heard. So if you find that happening, call out "Hard rules," meaning no one can speak until the speaker says your name, as though there is a talking stick in the room. The next person can only begin when the current speaker demarcates their conclusion by saying the next person's name. In essence, that is them handing over the talking stick. When done in large groups, the speaker will look to their right. Whoever wants to speak next raises their hand and the speaker will name whoever is closest to their right with their hand up. In a one-on-one conversation it's clear who is next, but in group settings, you go around to the right. Side note: This is especially useful in brainstorming sessions or when processing a contentious issue within a team. So if you're finding that you can't slow down, then agreeing to hard rules can cool down the rate of the exchange, creating the space for everyone to be heard.

Make Sure to Close the Space

If at any time either you or your partner want to stop the conversation because it has become too painful to continue, or simply time has run out and one of you has to leave, it is imperative that you close the space you opened when this conversation began. Do not simply end it when discomfort or conflict start to feel overwhelming. Instead, wherever you are in the conversation, stop, take a breath, and go to Questions 11 and 12. Ensuring that these final two questions are asked and answered will close the space on a connective note, no matter where it has taken you.

What to Do if You Feel Your Partner Isn't Fully Participating

It's not uncommon for one partner to feel excitement around entering into a conversation like this and for their partner to, well, not. They might see it as a trivial waste of time, or they might be terrified by the prospect of actively engaging in anything that would leave them feeling vulnerable. If that sounds like your partner but you're interested in having this conversation, be gentle and compassionate as you invite them into this experience with you. Remind them that they can utilize their pass if there's a question they don't want to answer for any reason. Reassure them that nothing specific needs to come out of the conversation and that no matter what happens, having the experience is what counts.

If you find that your partner is still hesitant to engage in this guided conversation with you, I'd suggest setting an appointed time to sit down and express to them how important it is to you that you play this game together and why. If they still refuse once you've told them you genuinely wish to have this experience, then perhaps it's time to consider what that tells you about your relationship. This is probably not the only instance in which you want to share something important to you with your partner and they are not meeting you in that space. That itself might be something constructive to start having a conversation about. At the end of the day, you can't force your partner into having this experience with you. Without the conscious and willing participation of both partners, you will not end up nurturing the kind of intimate connection these questions intend to develop.

Now, once you have both agreed to participate and have begun, if you feel that your partner is not committing as deeply to the emotional aspects of the conversation as you are or as you would like them to, take a step back and try to allow your partner the space to be who they are. You might be feeling that way because they simply aren't as skilled at emotional articulation as you are, and as we've seen, that can take practice. We all communicate in different ways and this may not be the way your partner communicates. They may communicate their emotions in other ways.

While this is an experience for you both to share, no one has to act a certain way, and there is no way to do it right other than to simply be in it. Soften your expectations and allow the conversation to unfold however it does naturally. If once you are done you feel it didn't reach the level of emotional depth you would have liked it to, remember that there is no such thing as perfect. We aren't even going for the "right" way. This is a practice of stepping into the space between and exploring what is present between you. You can always give it another go in the future, and the only sure thing is that each time will be different and reveal something new.

Where to Go from Here . . .

What if things go really, capital-B badly? What if by having this conversation you've realized that the connection between you and your partner isn't as strong as you thought—or might be completely untenable? Maybe they refuse to hear your truth. Or you realize that initial spark you used to feel has flickered and faded. Maybe, as happened in one of my relationships, you came to understand that you are simply on two different trajectories through life. Or, perhaps you realize for the very first time that the person you're sitting across from is actually nothing more and nothing less than a total and complete asshole. It happens.

So, what then? What if this conversation causes you and your partner to break up?

I won't lie to you—it's a possibility. I've seen it happen more than once. I remember being at a speaking engagement in Belgium and a fellow speaker approached me before I gave my talk.

"Hey, Topaz," he said to me without much preamble. "Those question cards of yours broke up my marriage!"

It's not uncommon for us to willfully ignore the places we don't resonate with our partner or where we have fallen out of resonance with them over time. Those out-of-tune notes simply don't sound nice. So we don't listen to them. We block them out. We might have invested so much in our relationship that sometimes we'd rather ignore the sound of dissonance than admit that we and our partners are no longer in harmony with each other. And even more importantly, confronting the fact that the will to find resonance has dissipated. Is that how we want to spend the rest of our lives? Turning down the volume on a song we no longer take full pleasure in? Wouldn't it be better to spend the brief time we have on earth fully immersed in a beautiful symphony, cranked up to full volume?

I've shared a lot about the importance of slowing down, of sitting in discomfort, of not rushing on to the next thing. I think this advice holds true in many situations, especially in the context of being actively engaged in the kind of conversations I am proposing. But every rule has its exceptions, and there are certainly times where it's unhelpful, even self-destructive, to be sitting in a painful situation any longer. Sometimes, moving on to our next chapter sooner rather than later is the best thing we can do.

I cut short what my fellow speaker said to me at that conference in Belgium. Yes, he did tell me that the questions I'd created broke up his marriage of many years. But do you know what the next thing he said to me was? He said, "Thank you. It helped me find the person I am with now. I am so much happier." And I could see in his eyes that he meant it.

If this conversation ends your relationship, that's great. Will that realization *feel* great in the moment? There's a good chance that it won't. But on an individual level, what more valuable resource do we have in life than our time? If this conversation helps you reach the end of a dissonant relationship quicker, aren't you that much closer to finding your next partner and learning the next lessons that they and the universe have in store for you? As we've seen again and again, one of the keys to a healthy relationship is the ability to handle the inevitable challenges and changes life will throw your way. If this conversation were one of those challenges and it couldn't be handled, I'd say that's very valuable information. If you find that your boat is leaky, that it can't handle the rocking of the waves, isn't your time better spent finding a new boat?

You could go on bailing out those leaks, exhausting yourself mentally and physically, for several more months or years. But do you really want to? Is that the best use of your time? Some leaks can absolutely be patched up once identified. But if you and your partner aren't going to patch the boat, meaning maintain it, then that doesn't bode well for the longevity of the boat.

All of that being said, statistically speaking this conversation is far more likely to bring you closer together than push you further apart. The vast majority of the hundreds and hundreds of couples I've seen engage with these questions have found that their level of intimacy blossomed far beyond what it had been. Their ability to weather storms increased and the lessons those storms offered became clearer. Their awareness of the teachings their partners offered them on a daily basis grew. And besides all of that, they had fun. They laughed, and when they cried they were grateful for their tears.

If you use the tools and fully give yourself over to your experience of stepping into the space between, this is the most likely outcome. But don't stop there. Even if your experience with these 12 questions goes better than you could have ever imagined, I still encourage you to come back to this conversation as many times as you see fit. Responses will change, your communication skills will get better and better, and your connection with your partner will grow ever stronger. Answering the final question I offer here isn't the end. In fact, I think you'll find it's quite the opposite.

CONCLUSIONS AND OTHER TAKEAWAYS

A few years ago, I packed my bags full of camera gear and made my way to Colorado's Western Slope. I was headed to a community of farmers, ranchers, and bona fide cowboys to make a film. As is usually the case whenever I venture out into the world to gather footage, I had no idea what I'd find there. Cows? Probably. Beautiful mountains? Hopefully. Dust? Most certainly. But beyond that, the canvas of my expectations was a perfect tabula rasa.

My time there ended up being one of the most fulfilling and educational experiences of my life for a whole host of reasons. Some of the things I learned at ten thousand feet altitude in the aspen-covered mountains were perfectly on brand for the cowboy-populated setting—lessons about responsibility, discipline, and how to model a healthy, positive masculine energy into my life. But perhaps the single most valuable teaching I received during my time in Colorado, which I cherish and try to practice to this day, was something I never would have guessed I'd discover amongst the cows, beautiful mountains, and dust that I did, indeed, find there in abundance: the secret to a successful marriage.

While I was filming, I had the great fortune to meet Carl and Joetta, a married couple of ranchers who call the Western Slope their home. From the first moment I met them, I was blown away by their connection, by the intimacy they carried with them into every moment of their every day. I spent a lot of time with them, enough to see them in various situations that ranged from the mundane to the tender to the tense. And that intimacy, that almost-tangible tether of love between them was always there, ever-mesmerizing. After days of this I had to ask: *What was their secret?* How had they cultivated a relationship that even to a stranger was so obviously thriving?

Like the generous and obliging people they proved themselves to be again and again, they told me. It was deceptively, almost comically, simple. Five nights a week at the very least, Carl and Joetta set aside an hour of their time. During this sacrosanct block of their evening, they pour each other a glass of wine, plop themselves into the hot tub in their backyard, gaze out at the Rocky Mountains, and talk about their lives and what they were experiencing. They would share their respective journeys, collectively and independently. It's the last bit that's the important part. The hot tub, the wine, the mountains—those are all nice, but they're not the secret—that would be the fact that Carl and Joetta intentionally, mindfully, and regularly set aside time to actively work on their connection via the art form of open and honest conversation. They've made a tradition out of it. I could see the fruits of that tradition in the way they looked at each other, in the way they disagreed, in their mutual respect. There is a deep love that's plainly, abundantly there for anyone who spends any amount of time with them to see.

Why do I bring them up here? Am I about to give you example questions pulled directly from their conversations for you to ask your partner? Am I about to try to sell you a hot tub or a membership to a wine club?

Of course not. Just as the scenery and the jacuzzi bubbles aren't what make Carl and Joetta's connection so special, I'd hazard a guess that it isn't really the specific content of their talks either. What makes their relationship so strong is the fact that they've made having conversations about their relationship into a practice, an act of maintenance they perform with joy and zeal on the regular. I can't stress enough how beneficial inviting healthy habits like this one into your relationship can be. Thus, simply said, *respect the date night.* Whether its once a week or five nights a week, make it a habit.

The conversation outlined in this book isn't something to just do once and forget about. Building intimate connections is a practice. I encourage you to come back to these questions and journey your way through the guided conversation they comprise as often as you like. Your responses will change and your connection with your partner will only become deeper the more you run through these powerful questions and others like them. I encourage you to move beyond the specific questions I've introduced in this book, augmenting your question inventory by using the tools you've learned here to start crafting better questions of your own. They won't just serve you well in your intimate relationships, but in every single connection you make with another human being over the course of your life. Let this book be the beginning of your practice of deepening all your relationships by asking better questions, even the relationship with yourself.

Building Yourself Better Questions

Think back to where we started, so many pages ago. I asked you to imagine the first moments of your day, to zero in on the thoughts that enter your mind in those bleary-eyed minutes, and to consider how each and every one of them is really the answer to a question you unconsciously ask yourself. If we are constantly asking ourselves questions, wouldn't bolstering the quality and thoughtfulness of those questions only add value, meaning, purpose, and joy to our lives? When it comes to the bigger questions, strengthening them in a few simple ways can greatly improve your quality of life.

By consciously asking yourself questions that have been crafted with the aim of bettering your quality of life and deepening your understanding of yourself—your decision-making, soul-searching, and personal development will all become both easier and more attuned with the person you truly are.

There are three parts to constructing a question when it comes to the ones we ask ourselves. The first is time frame. The second is how it affects you. The third is how it affects others.

Making the Infinite Finite

The first thing I'd suggest you consider when asking yourself a big question is giving it a clear, specific, and limited time frame in which to operate. When we're faced with an important decision, it can be easy to slip into the trap of thinking that said decision needs to apply forever. But remember, nothing is forever. Everything changes. Few decisions we can make are permanent, and embedding time periods into the questions you ask yourself acknowledges this fundamental rule of the universe. It also just makes the deciding process one heck of a lot less stressful.

Let's revisit a question my partner and I were asking ourselves at a pivotal moment of our lives. She and I were in the process of sorting out the particulars of where we wanted to raise our family, which, after she became pregnant with our second child, was about to expand. And so we asked: *Where do we want to live?* But, as I explained previously, that question didn't offer a clear answer. And so our question became, *Where do we want to live for the next year, until our new baby is six months old, that will support us in creating a nurturing and loving environment for our young children and inspire us to give more of ourselves to one another?*

What was the first change to the wording of that question?

. . . for the next year, until our new baby is six months old . . .

That was the first puzzle piece that, when it fell into place, made our decision so much easier to make. We weren't staring down the barrel of the rest of our lives, trying to figure out where we wanted to put down permanent, intractable roots. We just had to think about what place we wanted to be in for the next year. That was all. And that was much more manageable to wrap our minds around.

Let Your Feelings Guide You

If we continue to break down the strengthened version of *Where do we want to live?* we come to . . . *and inspire us to give more of ourselves to one another.* This part of the question was helpful for us because it tapped into the way a potential answer to this question would directly affect how we'd feel. When we were looking for a new home, my partner and I started to think about how we, personally, wanted to feel in that place. After a bit of self-reflection, we decided we wanted to feel inspired, and be allowed to feel like our most loving selves. Just like with the time limit, this narrowed down the options. It made finding an answer easier. But it also helped us really focus on what we *actually* wanted out of our home. Asking a better question helped us do that in a way that *Where do we want to live?* never could have.

Taking the Ripple Effect into Account

Here is the last change we made to the question that guided us to find and feel comfortable in our home: *that will support us in creating a nurturing and loving environment for our young children.*

We had to acknowledge that the answer to our question wasn't just going to affect either of us individually. Like any decision we make in our lives, it was going to affect the people around us. We wanted to feel like the place itself was nurturing our family. And that's the final aspect of creating better questions to ask yourself: consider the ripple effects it will have on your community and vice versa.

Developing Your Own Questions

These building blocks will not only help you create self-directed questions from scratch, but you can also shape a question to your needs and then see what possibilities emerge. This is more empowering, exciting, and most importantly, places you in a position of agency. Let's take a look at a few examples.

What job should I get? That's a question that I think a lot of us ask, whether we're looking for our first job or next job. There's clearly an opportunity here to improve this self-inquiry. First, let's just give it a time frame. Maybe changing it to *What job should I pursue for the next chapter in my career?* will help take some of the pressure off. It's just the next chapter. It's a next step, nothing more.

Now let's infuse the question with our second element for crafting better questions: How you feel about it. How about, *What job would inspire me for the next chapter in my career?* Or maybe one of the following options feels best for you: *What am I most passionate about for the next chapter of my career? What job would excite me the most for the next chapter of my career? What job am I scared to aim for and yet excites me for the next chapter of my career? What job would be the biggest challenge for me for the next chapter of my career? What job is most strategic for the next step in my career?* You could fill in different adjectives and ideas around how you might feel in that job or how that job might affect you.

Now, let's add in the layer of how it affects the people around you. In this case—*What job would inspire me for the next chapter in my career?*—you could tweak it to become *What job would inspire me for the next chapter that would allow me to* [fill in the blank; that is, *to contribute most to my industry, to support my family in this time of challenge,* or *inspire others to follow suit to tackle the biggest challenges that I feel need to be addressed in this day and age*]. Whatever it is, you can see that by playing with these three components to a question, different possibilities emerge. Your mind is incredible at finding answers. Be sure you are giving it wonderful questions to solve.

Another example question: *Why am I not in the shape I want to be in?* Already you can see how that question is constructed to lead you down a troubled path. You can only get negative answers from this question. Instead of *Why am I not in the shape I want to be in?*

we could give it a more empowering perspective by adding the time frame so it says, *What can I do for the next three weeks to get into better shape?* We're already making it more positive by adding *What can I do,* so you're looking for places of action. And you give yourself a manageable time frame—the next three weeks—in which to put those ideas into action.

Now let's refine and deepen this question. What does "better shape" actually mean? That is too broad. Let's focus on how it makes you feel: *What can I do for the next three weeks that will enable me to feel more vital and invigorated?* Now you're asking yourself to generate empowering solutions and ideas, within a time frame, and with a clear idea of how the answer will affect you.

And now we will add the third layer, which is how it affects other people. So, what if the question becomes *What can I do for the next three weeks that will enable me to feel more vital and invigorated such that I can engage more with my kids when I play with them?* Or . . . *so that I can take my kids on a three-hour hike?* This way you can really hone in on a more wonderful, tangible, inspiring answer than what the original question *Why am I not in the shape I want to be in?* would get you—a question that is empowering, one that is achievable because it has a time frame, and one that connects you to other people and has a positive impact on them.

What about the question *How am I ever going to come back from this?* When really bad things happen, this might be one of the questions you try to answer. What if we changed this question to *What does mental and emotional health look like for me a year from now?* This way we're clarifying what "coming back from this" means— emotional and mental health—and giving it a time frame. And we can dig even deeper. If we want an answer to *What does mental and emotional health actually feel like for me?* why don't we tweak it to *What does feeling fulfilled and joyful look like for me a year from now?* See how just adjusting the element of how something feels for you can lead you in a different direction?

Now let's add the last layer of having an effect on other people, leaving us with the question *In a year from now, what does it look like for me to feel fulfilled and joyful so that I'm in a position to positively support my loved ones?* Or *How can I achieve a sense of fulfillment and joy, so that in a year from now I will be able to share my journey with others going through a similar predicament?* By giving a question a time frame, we are keeping it tangible and accessible. By stating how it makes us feel and how it affects others, we are both clarifying what the possible answer could be and also giving us motivation to follow through.

The idea here is to play and explore the three facets to a question. Continue to replace the three aspects to any question with different possibilities and then see what feels best. Where does it lead you? Do you feel more empowered, with more agency and capability than before? This is what I mean by stop searching for answers, create better questions. Use more creativity in creating the question and you will find a more powerful, empowering answer.

The Point of It All

The exercise of asking yourself better questions doesn't just make the act of finding an answer easier; it fundamentally changes your experience of life and your perception and representation of the world around you. Becoming more aware of the way your decisions affect your feelings by baking this consideration into your questions can allow you to clearly see what works and what doesn't for you on your lifelong journey toward fulfillment, growth, expansion, and deepening. It brings agency into how you construct meaning in your life. Asking questions that take the people around you into account will naturally lead you to see the interconnectedness that we all share as human beings—the same species living on the same planet. And constantly reminding yourself that time in a precious and limited quantity can serve as a reminder that all things end, thus syncing up your thinking with the natural flow of life.

So rather than asking the question *Is this the person I want to be with forever?* ask *Is this the person I want to spend the next few chapters of my life with? Someone with whom I can embark on a journey of growth and learning that will enrich us both until that chapter ends?* Now that's a question to be proud of, one that honors the truth in you, the truth in your partner, and the truth of the universe. Because all chapters end. The only constant in life is change and the only sure thing about it is that one day we'll die. However, I can't think of a better way to spend the time we do have on Earth than consciously building intimate, vibrant, and meaningful connections with the people we share that time with. Doing this—and doing it fully, bravely, vulnerably—is what makes life worth living. It can even make that moment of confronting the reality that all things end a sweet and beautiful experience.

Final Thoughts: Interpersonal Connection Is Universal

In 1995 I had the extreme privilege of visiting two Indigenous tribes deep in the Amazon rainforest. I spent two weeks with the Asurini and Araweté tribes, which Western civilization had only come into contact with in 1979 and 1981, respectively. One night with the Asurini, I was invited to a healing ceremony for an elder nearing the end of her life. I peeked in at the entrance of the large hut. A strong smell of tobacco and smoke filled a space that fit almost twenty people. In the center of the hut was a fire and a shaman. Beside the shaman was an old woman, basically skin and bones in her hammock. You could barely make her out but for her luminescent eyes reflecting the fire and the scene around her. Surrounding her in concentric circles was her family. Starting with other elders from her generation and extending all the way through her children, now adults, and their partners, to her grandchildren littering the edge of the lodging, seemingly unaware of the passing that was about to transpire. As the shaman sang and did his work, I was captivated by the way this old woman was staring at her friends, children, and grandchildren. This was her community over time. And although she was too weak to move or speak, her eyes shone with a brilliant intensity as she looked at them. It was clear to me that she was finding peace and even joy in her final moments because of the connection she had developed with her loved ones over the course of her life. How many of us will have such a loving transition into death? How many of us will see our relationships echo into the future with such grace and kindness?

The importance of our interpersonal connections is universal. It transcends culture and even time. Building these connections is a lasting gift that we can give each other and ourselves. The more tightly our stories are intertwined with those of the people we are closest with, the happier and healthier we'll be. And the act of sharing those stories with one another, through something as simple as conversation, can be nothing less than medicine.

What gifts has your life experience shaped such that you can offer them to others? I've received many gifts in my life that I've tried, in my small way, to pass on to you. My parents' divorce, my long and arduous quest for intimacy, the countless hours witnessing people sharing their vulnerabilities with one another, the joy and learning {THE AND} has brought into my life—these were all gifts that I was given by life that I now offer to you here, as stories and, hopefully, as medicine. Search your past, your present, and look to your future for your own gifts. What life experiences have bestowed you with gifts that you can now share with others? Pass them on to those around you as often as you can. If we do this, the world can become that much more of a loving place.

Ultimately don't fear the pain or discomfort. Embrace it. Embrace it especially with those you love. Love is a practice. How can we indulge in it if we don't step into the space between?

ACKNOWLEDGMENTS

First and foremost, I want to give a heartfelt thank-you to all {THE AND} participants. My team and I created the space and the platform to hear and share your stories, but ultimately it is you, the participants, who stepped in with courage to share your vulnerabilities and relationships with us. {THE AND} as a film project or this book would be nothing without you. You are the fundamental kernel from which this project grew and all the learnings garnered. A heartful thank-you.

To those who walked the path of building The Skin Deep as an experience design studio with me. There are too many names to fit all here, but key contributors who offered not just their time but their hearts too, include Nicholas D'Agostino, Julia Gorbach, Carla Tramullas, Chris Mcnabb, Dane Benko, Meriem Dehbi Talbot, Nazareth Soberanes, Candice Frazer, Heran Abate, Alison Goerke, Alvaro Garza Rios, Anndi Liggett, Ashika Kuruvilla, Bojana Ceranic, Chelsea Weber, Fernando Espinosa Vera, Kat Hennessey, Rosie Gardel, Grace Larkin, Hans Leuders, Jaydin Lopez, Levy Toredjo, Melanie Rosette, Nick Dunlap, Paige Polk, Rebecca Diaz, Sydney Laws, Julian Dario Villa, and Tyler Rattray. To the many long hours worked and the beautiful challenges overcome, I am grateful to you for your contribution and commitment.

To Nathan Phillips, Lior Levy, Jeremiah and Noemie Zagar, Jacob Bronstein, Richard Tripp, Christian Contreras, Jun Harada, Mike Knowlton, Mark Harris, Lindsey Cordero, Anthony Cabraal, Armando Croda, Justin Thomson, Tracey Smith, Adrian Belic, Jarrin Kirksey, Brian Fountain, Peter Riedel, Camillia BenBassat, Tricia Neves, Thomas Droge, Kevin Courtney, Lilianna Legge, Rich Bodo, Andrew Hoppin, Gabriel Noble, Marjan Tehrani, Paola Mendoza, Michael and Martha

Skolnik; thank you for your treasured advice and contribution over the years to The Skin Deep and all its projects. Your hearts are as big as your insights. I am grateful to you for offering both to me on the journey over the last ten years.

There are a group of people that have supported me from day one as a twenty-four-year-old filmmaker and my twenty-three-year journey since. They have offered financial support when I needed it most, harsh advice when it was imperative I hear it, and a place to find solace when I didn't know where to turn. Kristoph Lodge, Ersin Akarlilar, Ben Edwards, Santiago Dellepiane, Shoham Adizes, Dana and Danny Gabriel, Jonathan Price, Adam Somner, Carmen Ruiz de Huidobro, and Ivan Saldana. Your resolute belief in me has been the buttress against doubt and challenges in all its forms and without which nothing I envisioned would come to pass. Thank you for being my pillar.

To my mentors Tom Sturgess, Donny and Jackie Epstein, Nathaniel D. R., Tamahau Rowe, Pekaira Rei, Erik Kolbell, and Ramses Erdtmann. You have shined the light before me even when I didn't want to look. You expanded my understanding of what's possible and how to get there. And most importantly you have taught me the valuable, hard lessons of what it means to be human stepping into the responsibility of offering all of oneself to something bigger.

To our publishing team of Tony Ong (designer), Isabella Hardie (production editor), Melat Ermyas (intern), and Jen Worick (publisher), who have made this process an absolute joy. To Jill Saginario, the wonderful editor of this project, your resolute perspective has been the keel of this journey constantly moving us forward in line to our envisioned destination. To Ben Grenrock, your commitment and talent in contributing to the words in this book and clarifying the structure of the ideas in it are simply invaluable. To Zander Blunt, thank you for pressing me on the concepts presented and the ways of communicating them. To Juan Jorge García Mendez, thank you for offering me a beautiful, calm space in which to dive deep into my work of the last ten years and write this book. And a kind appreciation to Eric Rayman, my literary lawyer and experienced guide through the publishing world.

To Sonya Renee Taylor, thank you for your beautiful words in the foreword, and in sharing your life story with me for the last six years. I honor not only your path but more importantly the love and faith in which you walk it. We are soul siblings and I treasure every time we share the trail notes of our lives.

To my parents and siblings, thank you for being who you are. Tria, Ichak, Nurit, Shoham, Atalia, Nimrod, Cnaan, and Sapphire, you are the family unit that shaped the person I am today and I come from that space of intimacy we all have shared together. To my wife's family in Mexico, you have welcomed me in with the warmest of hearts and kind generosity of which I am eternally grateful and blessed to be a part of.

Finally and most importantly, to Icari, my life partner, you are the greatest thing that has ever happened to me. Everything blossoms from the grace of your love. Thank you for teaching me the essential experience of intimacy and continuously practicing with me the art of love. To my two children, Cosmos and Lylah Oceana, I hope that one day this book will help you as you venture out upon your own path of intimacy, love, and connection.

FURTHER QUESTIONS

QUESTION 1: What are your three favorite memories we share and why do you cherish them? (page 56)

- When was the first time you knew I loved you?
- When was the first time you knew you loved me?
- What's the craziest thing I've done for our love?
- What is something you would never have done if it wasn't for me?
- If for some reason I lost my memory, what's the first thing you'd tell me about us?

QUESTION 2: What was your first impression of me and how has that changed over time? (page 64)

- Describe what our first meeting was like, but from my perspective.
- If you could go back to when we first met, what advice would you give yourself in terms of being in a relationship with me?
- What do you think I remember most from our first meeting and why?
- What do you think has shaped me the most to be ready for this relationship and why?

QUESTION 3: When do you feel closest to me and why? (page 72)

- What do you feel connects us?
- What do you believe is unique about our relationship?
- What makes us, us?
- What's your favorite imperfection of mine and why?
- What do I do that you love that I'm not aware of?
- What do I do that makes you love me more?

QUESTION 4: What are you hesitant to tell me and why? (page 81)

- What do you think I am hesitant to ask you and why?
- What do you think I am hesitant to tell you and why?
- What are you hesitant to ask me and why?
- What's your biggest concern that you haven't shared with me before?
- What do you feel we avoid talking about and why do you think that is?

QUESTION 5: What is the biggest challenge in our relationship right now and what do you think it is teaching us? (page 93)

- Where do you believe there is room for growth in our relationship?
- What in your opinion can I do to improve our relationship and why?
- What's currently missing from our relationship and what can we do to change that?
- What's been the biggest challenge for us as a couple recently, and what did we learn about each other in overcoming it?

QUESTION 6: What is a sacrifice you feel you've made that I haven't acknowledged and why do you think that is? (page 105)

- When was the time I disappointed you most and how do you feel about it now?
- What's been the hardest thing for you that I didn't see or understand?
- What is something you feel I still don't understand about you and why do you think that is?
- What do you need from me and am I providing it?

QUESTION 7: What is the pain in me you wish you could heal and why? (page 114)

- When do you worry about me most and why?
- What's a mistake you see me make repeatedly and why do you think I do?
- How would I be able to heal from the pain I went through, while being with you, and without you?
- What's an experience you wish I never had and what do you think it taught me?

QUESTION 8: What is one experience you wish we never had and why? (page 124)

- What in your opinion is the experience that has shaped us the most and why?
- What do you think we avoid the most and what can we do about it?
- When was the last time you considered ending this relationship, and why didn't you?
- What was our worst fight and what did it teach you about loving me?

QUESTION 9: What do you think you're learning from me? (page 134)

- How have I changed you?
- When do you admire me most that I'm not aware of?
- Why do you think I am in your life?
- What have you learned about me this year that makes you love me more?
- What's my superpower that I'm not aware of?
- When have you seen me at my most vulnerable and what has it taught you about loving me?

QUESTION 10: What is one experience you can't wait for us to share and why? (page 143)

- What do you see for us in the next five years?
- If you could wish one thing for me, what would it be and why?
- If you could grant us any three wishes, what would it be and why?

QUESTION 11: If this was our last conversation, what would you never want me to forget? (page 153)

- What's something you think I need to hear and why?
- What do you think life is teaching me right now and why?
- What do you think life has brought us together for?

QUESTION 12: Why do you love me? (page 164)

- What does my love feel like?
- How do I love you?
- What do you find most beautiful about my love?
- What do you find most beautiful about my love that I may not be aware of?

REFERENCES

If you would like to view the moments referred to in the book, scan the QR code and it will take you there.

Introduction

Rafa & Douglas •
"Polyamorous and
Monogamous Love"

The Tools

Curtis & John • "A Son Confesses to His Father"	Sidra & Ben • "One of Our Hardest Times"	Sidra & Ben • "Compilation"

Question 1: What are your three favorite memories we share and why do you cherish them?

Kat & Christina •
"How Does Deafness
Affect Our Family?"

Question 2: What was your first impression of me and how has that changed over time?

Cat & Keith •
"A Major Transition"

"How Couples Found
Their Love Together"

"What Do You
Remember From
When We Met?"

Question 3: When do you feel closest to me and why?

Maddi & Martin •
"The Pain in Me You'd
Like to Heal"

Watch a compilation
video for this
question.

Question 4: What are you hesitant to ask me and why?

Sidra & Ben • "How
a Baby Can Change
Your Marriage"

Ivo & Kevin •
"Balancing Love &
Anxiety in Marriage"

Andrew & Jerrold •
"Gay Marriage & My
Religious Family"

Watch a compilation
video for this
question.

Question 5: What is the biggest challenge in our relationship right now and what do you think it is teaching us?

Gabrielle & Luna •
"Friends Trying
to Confess Their
Romantic Feelings"

Watch a compilation
video for this
question.

Question 6: What is a sacrifice you feel you've made that I haven't acknowledged and why do you think that is?

Kat & Christina •
"How Does Deafness
Affect Our Family?"

Ivo & Kevin •
"Balancing Love &
Anxiety in Marriage"

Watch a compilation
video for this
question.

Question 7: What is the pain in me you wish you could heal and why?

Maddi & Martin •
"The Pain in Me You'd
Like to Heal"

Lynnea & Eliza • "I'm
Gonna NOT Answer
That Question"

Andrew & Jerrold •
"Gay Marriage & My
Religious Family"

Question 8: What is one experience you wish we never had and why?

Sidra & Ben • "How
to Fall Back in Love"

Marcela & Rock •
"Most Honest Couple
on Earth"

Question 9: What do you think you are learning from me?

Andrew & Jerrold •
"Gay Marriage & My
Religious Family"

Andrew & Jerrold •
"Gay Marriage & My
Religious Family"
continued

**Question 10: What is one experience you can't wait for us to
share and why?**

Ikeranda & Josette •
"Building a Blended
Family as a Same-
Gender Couple"

Keisha & Andrew •
"I Wanna Take Care
of You"

Keisha & Andrew •
"Would You Confront
the Racists in Your
Family?"

Question 11: If this was our last conversation, what would you never want me to forget?

Kelly & Virgie •
"If I Left This Earth
Tomorrow"

Watch a compilation
video for this
question.

Question 12: Why do you love me?

Marcela & Rock •
"Most Honest Couple
on Earth"

Rafa & Douglas •
"Polyamorous and
Monogamous Love"

Watch a compilation
video for this
question.

ABOUT THE AUTHOR

TOPAZ ADIZES is an Emmy award-winning writer, director, and experience design architect. He is an Edmund Hillary fellow and Sundance/Skoll stories of change fellow. His works have been selected to Cannes, Sundance, IDFA, and SXSW; featured in *New Yorker* magazine, *Vanity Fair*, and the *New York Times*; and have garnered an Emmy for new approaches to documentary and two World Press Photo awards for immersive storytelling and interactive documentary. He is currently the founder and executive director of the experience design studio The Skin Deep. Topaz studied philosophy at UC Berkeley and Oxford University. He speaks four languages, and currently lives in Mexico with his wife and two children.

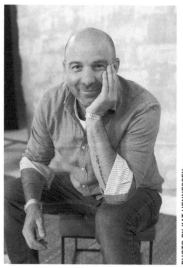

PHOTO BY KAT HENNESSEY

For more about The Skin Deep, visit TheSkinDeep.com.

To learn more about Topaz Adizes and his work, visit TopazAdizes.com.